CRACKING THE DISEASE CODE

Revealing Disease Causes, from Spiritual to Physical

Darius Soon

Published: December 2016

ISBN: 978-981-11-0901-0

Rights

Conditions of Sale

Disclaimer

This book is not to be considered medical advice. Your circumstances and characteristics — physical, emotional, mental and spiritual — are unique to you; I don't know what they are, and cannot offer any advice on them.

Do your own independent research into the information in this book before accepting anything. If you do follow the advice in this book, please take personal responsibility for the outcomes. The author and publisher cannot take medical or legal responsibility for any consequences arising from your following this advice.

With regard to case studies used in this book, we have made every effort to conceal the identity of all individuals in order to preserve their privacy. To this end, all names, physical descriptions, professions and even the gender have been changed.

Printed by ColourXpress Printing Pte Ltd

CONTENTS

TEN — Past Lives: You have Lived Before 165

ELEVEN — Spirits: Death is Not the End 177

PREFACE

"You never know how much you really believe anything until its truth or falsehood becomes a matter of life and death to you."

C. S. Lewis

It took me a long time to decide to write this book. The reason is simple: its contents go against the grain of many people's beliefs. I therefore expect a fair amount of criticism and skepticism, especially since I was never formally trained in medicine or health care. In fact, by formal education I am an accountant.

However, I also know that for people suffering from major, chronic, life-threatening diseases, this book can be a matter of life and death. Withholding this information would therefore be criminal.

I have thus decided to allow the contents to speak for themselves. You of course are free to draw your own conclusions about the validity of this work. Most importantly, I hope to create a dialogue and discussion about the true causes of disease, without pre-conceived notions and dogma clouding the issues.

My name is Darius Soon, and I am a medical intuitive. A medical intuitive can sense the physical conditions affecting a person, the true cause for these conditions, and propose solutions to make the person better — all, usually, without ever even seeing the person.

I'll now briefly recount how I went from being an auditor in one of the then Big Five accounting firms to being a medical intuitive.

I was sensitive even as a child and growing up in practical-minded Singapore was tough. Despite my spiritual inclinations, I took

Preface

what was considered the 'secure' route when it came to my career: I enrolled myself in Nanyang Business School, Nanyang Technological University.

After graduating with high honors, I started work as an auditor in the prestigious audit firm of PricewaterCoopers. I found being an auditor a soul-wrecking business. When I finished my first year in the firm and saw the results of my work — rows and rows of audited accounts — I wasn't the least bit thrilled about the 'difference I had made'.

It was time for some re-evaluation, and I tread the route many youths facing a quarter-life crisis do: I took a sabbatical of close to a year to travel round the world. During that journey, my best experience bar none was a two-week stint as a volunteer in Kripalu Yoga Centre near Boston. During those two weeks, one of the most fascinating lectures I attended was by a lady who used *Reiki*, a form of hands-on healing, to treat people with different types of illnesses. I was fascinated enough to want to learn it myself when I returned to Singapore.

During my travels, it also dawned on me that how I was behaving with others was pushing them away. I had always known something was wrong with my interaction with others; somewhere along the way on this long trip, I found the label for it: low self-esteem.

This low self-esteem formed the core of my personality then, and manifested itself in different ways.

For example, I had difficulties with authority. I couldn't speak up or voice my opinions even when I believed my views to be right. I took a torturous amount of time to make decisions simply because I often had to consider whether my decision would please everyone else. I often subconsciously compared myself with others and found myself coming up short.

This created a huge dent in my confidence with girls or in my job. It was almost as if I had an inner voice berating me constantly for never being good enough. I started looking for solutions.

Before my round-the-world-find-myself trip, I had spent three years studying with a Zen teacher who had been endorsed by a *Roshi* (literally 'teacher') in Japan for having had some enlightenment experiences. She was however having conflicts with her husband and they were on the verge of divorcing.

My Zen teacher went for a seminar that used energy psychology to treat how she felt. After that session, her issues with her husband resolved themselves, and she became a fervent supporter of the approach. She advised me to give it a go.

At first, I was very skeptical, but what changed my mind were the changes I saw in Phoebe. Phoebe was one of the students in my class. Phoebe and I were the 'outsiders' in the class; while the others would gather around after meditation for small talk, Phoebe and I invariably found ourselves in a corner, sitting next to each other.

Phoebe agreed to go for the energy psychology seminar. The following week, at our meditation session, Phoebe didn't join me in our usual corner. Instead, she joined the others and began chatting happily away as if she had been doing that all along. It was like she became a whole new person.

Intrigued, I found myself at the same seminar a few weeks later. By the end of that seminar, I had felt a huge shift within myself.

The night after that seminar, I was having dinner with my course mates. To my great surprise, I found myself in animated conversation with them instead of being my usual shy and quiet self. When I caught myself doing so, I went "Wow, what has happened to me?"

When my self-esteem — something that had plagued me for over twenty years — could disappear in one day, the natural question to ask was, "What am I missing?" Obviously something profound had happened.

Over the next ten years, I would dedicate my life to finding out what energy psychology and energy medicine was all about.

Along the way, I started working with people with all sorts of emotional issues: grief, phobias, self-esteem issues, procrastination and others. I discovered that emotions had a strong link to disease. I saw firsthand how working with and resolving negative emotions that someone had felt for a long time could turn around a physical condition as well.

I started a business using energy healing to work with autistic children. Some autistic children improved remarkably within a short span of three months, while others didn't seem to see any change in that period (though I would later find out that some of the latter did improve over a much longer period). The huge inconsistency in results over the first three months unsettled me.

I needed a roadmap of health and disease — and I found it in the teachings of Dr. Dietrich Klinghardt, MD.

Dr. Klinghardt provided a comprehensive framework comprising five levels of healing and his Autonomic Response Testing (ART) tool for the causes and appropriate intervention for physical illnesses. Using his ART I developed my own Medical Intuition System (MIS), an energy-scanning technique that allows me to know what is happening in the body of a person, as well as the causes and solutions, by accessing her energy field.

Then something uncanny happened. Through a series of coincidences, I was given guardianship over a gateway that allows me to send spirits over to the 'other realms'. At first, I didn't understand the implications of having this gateway.

One of the things I learned from Dr. Klinghardt was that a bacterium is responsible for Lyme disease, and it seems to pop up in everyone with chronic illness. It takes many years to deal with this bacterium.

Around that time, a mother with an 18-year-old autistic teen came to see me. While I was working with the teen, I discovered that he had a spirit 'attached' to him. I sent the spirit off through the gateway I controlled and then found out, to my great surprise, that I could no longer detect the Lyme bacterium energy on him!

This gave me a profound realization: spirits are responsible for creating a distortion in a person's energy field that then leads to the growth of virulent bacteria. Removing the spirits allows the body to start detoxing and coming back to balance in the most effective way.

That insight changed my practice completely. I started to focus on addressing these spirit attachments in my clients. The moment I started doing that, I started seeing both greater consistency of results and a plunge in the number of sessions needed for recovery, although there are cases of clients who take a longer time to respond to the therapies.

Later on in the book I introduce a concept known as the *morphogenetic field*. Different people have called this field by different names: auras, the Akashic records, etc. Call it what you like.

Preface

All the names refer to the same thing: the memories of everything that has ever happened to a person.

By tapping into this information, which I now do on a regular basis with my clients, I have seen common patterns that seem to lie at the heart of a person's disease or condition. Accessing this information has allowed me to realize that there are many misconceptions about diseases that are currently held as truth in the medical and health establishment.

I completely understand if you find it difficult to believe in a process that involves tapping into invisible fields. One way to establish the truth of the ideas I'm asserting is to search for independent sources from different authorities, and see whether these sources have come to similar conclusions regarding these ideas.

I myself did this and was pleasantly surprised to find that these very different sources do in fact converge on the same explanations.

This book is divided into two parts:
1. Part I, where I discuss why medicine is due for a renewal;
2. Part II, where I discuss the Traumatic Memories as Source of Disease (TMSD) model, the model that I am proposing will help crack the disease code and explain what I believe are the true causes for disease. This model differs substantially from the mainstream view, held by conventional medical professionals or within *allopathic* (generally Western) medicine, as the causes for diseases.

Preface

Some of what I write may sound incredible. All I am asking for is an open-minded attitude and a willingness to seek the truth yourself.

"If it's not broken, don't fix it."

That's the conventional adage. Indeed, if our medical system were perfect, this book would never have been written.

In Part I of the book, I go into some of the flaws in our current, conventional paradigm of health, and why they exist. Part I comprises three chapters:

a. In Chapter One, I discuss the scientific method as it's currently practiced and why the information in this book is not well known to the public.

b. In Chapter Two, I talk about the principles underlying the approach that allopathic medicine uses to treat disease, and explore their effectiveness in achieving that goal.

c. In Chapter Three, I go into the problem of consciousness and show how allopathic medicine, by ignoring consciousness, can never get to the true root causes of illnesses.

Readers who do not wish to understand, or are already familiar with, allopathic medicine's model and flaws can go directly to Part II where I lay the groundwork for the TMSD model that I believe reveals the spiritual to physical causes of disease.

Part II consists of 12 chapters:

d. In Chapter Four, I explain how all disease is ultimately linked to stress.

e. In Chapter Five, I discuss traumas, and the traumas-stress-disease link.

f. In Chapter Six, current-life traumas are explored, including birth and childhood memories and how they can affect our health.

g. In Chapter Seven, I cover the mechanism of memories — the bridge between traumas and stress — by showing how past traumatic incidents can still continue to bring about stress in the current moment. I also explore what memories are all about and where they are stored.

h. In Chapter Eight, myths about genes are unraveled.

i. In Chapter Nine, I talk about how epigenetics and traumas experienced by our ancestors can still continue to haunt us today.

j. In Chapter Ten, I go into the controversial topic of past lives, ie whether reincarnation exists and how events from these past lives can affect our current life.

k. In Chapter Eleven, the controversial topic of spirits, and how these spirits can be responsible for all disease, is covered.

l. In Chapter Twelve, I backtrack and cover why germs are not responsible for our illnesses.

m. In Chapter Thirteen, I cover the most common lifestyle factors often mentioned as being linked to disease — the foods we eat, how much exercise we do — and explore whether these are the true causes of our ailments.

n. In Chapter Fourteen, I look at other environmental factors, and explore how our consciousness can potentially shape our environment to cause health or illness.

o.   In Chapter Fifteen, I relate how we are all part of a much bigger system that includes the Earth and the Sun, and how diseases are ultimately linked to imbalances in our relationships with these larger systems.

Finally, in the Conclusion, I bring all these different principles together to Crack the Disease Code. Let's begin!

INTRODUCTION — Perspectives: How Sometimes It May Not Be 'Either-Or' But 'And'

The year was 1791.

Fredrich Nicolai, a German writer, was suffering from giddiness. The year before, he had missed his twice-a-year appointment with his physician for routine 'bloodletting' (a procedure in which leeches are placed on the skin to drain out 'excess' blood). It was believed that this procedure re-established the balance of 'vital humors' (where humors refer to blood, bile and fluids) which helped to restore health. Those days it was standard medical practice to treat giddiness in this manner.

One morning, while under extreme stress, Fredrich was shocked to encounter a ghost in his room. His wife couldn't see it, but he could. With each passing week he began seeing more ghosts. This went on for a few weeks. Apparently, they were trying to communicate with him. As the situation worsened, he decided to meet his physician and have him do the usual ritual of bloodletting. The outcome? His 'hallucinations' began to fade.

After this incident, Fredrich concluded that what had happened to him could happen to anyone. The cure was to balance one's humors through bleeding. He wrote an article about the incident that was highly commended by the medical establishment of the day for its rationality and objectivity.[1]

Introduction - Perspectives: How Sometimes It May Not Be 'Either-Or' But 'And'

However, had any *shamans* — healers, typically from northern Asia and North America, thought to have access to the world of good and evil spirits — been around to consider Fredrich's case, they would immediately have concluded that Fredrich was disturbed by troubled spirits.

Their solution would have been to perform a proper ritual to appease the spirits. They would have proclaimed that the spirits had been around him all the time, but he had been able to see them only when his body had been significantly 'out of balance'. Being around these spirits for a prolonged period could also have been the cause of his giddiness.

Now let's consider the same scenario in modern times. Fredrich would visit a psychiatrist who would conclude that these hallucinations were the effect of an imbalance in *neurotransmitters* (like dopamine and serotonin), the current dominant view in biomedicine. Fredrich would be diagnosed with symptoms of psychosis or schizophrenia and prescribed lifelong haloperidol medication.

So which era had the right perspective in determining the cause of the disease? Was it the shamanic view: the taking into account of the possibility of supernatural influences? Or was the medieval perspective — balancing of humors as the way to good health — right? Or would modern times, where only a biomedical view of health is considered, be correct?

This is similar to a well-known fable. Three blind men feel three different parts of an object (an elephant), and each conclude the object to be a different thing.

Introduction - Perspectives: How Sometimes It May Not Be 'Either-Or' But 'And'

The blind man who touched the tusk of the elephant described what he'd touched as a sharp object; the man who caressed the trunk thought it was a snake; and the man who had touched the feet declared the object to be a tree. None could understand that he'd touched an elephant albeit a different part of it.

Using this analogy, perhaps all three beliefs — shamanic, medieval and biomedical — were correct, just seen from different viewpoints. The right perspective to adopt here may not be 'either or' but an inclusive 'and'.

In this book, I would like to explore the possibility that all these views are valid, and thus transform the way we think about the true causes of diseases.

"All truth passes through three stages. First, it is ridiculed. Second, it is violently opposed. Third, it is accepted as being self-evident."
Arthur Schopenhauer

PART I
WHY MEDICINE IS
DUE FOR A
RENEWAL

ONE — Science: Science Advances through Anomalies

Anomalies are the Keys to a New Paradigm

When Sir Isaac Newton came up with his theory of Newtonian mechanics and James Clerk Maxwell finalized his equations describing electromagnetic waves, it was believed that physics was finally complete. Lord Kelvin said in 1900, "There is nothing new to be discovered in physics now, all that remains is more and more precise measurement."[2]

Yet, by the 1900s, scientists had begun to observe slight differences between results predicted by the Newtonian model and results actually observed for gravity, especially when looking at the orbit of planets like Mercury around the Sun. It was not until Albert Einstein revolutionized the idea of space-time in his general theory of relativity in 1915 that this discrepancy was explained.[3]

Intuitively, we would think that all Einstein did was to take Newton's law of gravity and modify it. But that wasn't what happened. Far from it: he had to create the model anew. Newton saw gravity as two masses pulling upon each other. However, Einstein discovered that space itself contains a shape, and space and time are inextricably linked, hence the term 'space-time'.

Space-time can be likened to a spider web with an object placed on it. Any object with sufficient mass (for our purposes here, read 'mass' as 'weight') will cause the web to sag, tightening around the area where the object is located and creating a depression in the web. The bigger and heavier the object, the bigger the depression created in the web.

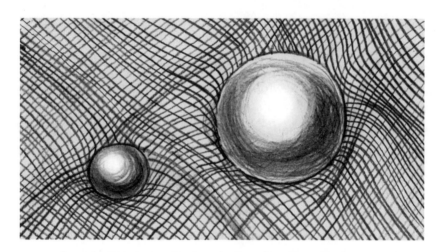

Figure 1: Space-Time Curvature Illustrated

If two objects are placed side-by-side on the spider web, the web will sag in two places, making the objects appear closer. To an external observer who cannot see the web it would look like the two objects are pulling upon each other, when it is the space around the two objects that has become warped causing the objects to move towards each other.

Einstein's model was able to explain all the problems that Newton's law of gravitation could *plus* everything that the Newtonian model couldn't.

That, fundamentally, is how theories in science should evolve. There is an anomaly that doesn't fit the standard norms and rules of how things work. Someone comes up with a radical hypothesis that can fit all the data sets more completely, thereby indicating that this new conjecture is more in touch with reality than the previous paradigm. It is also likely that this new paradigm is not just a simple modification of the previous concept, but a substantial overhaul of it.

Science However is Rejecting Anomalies

Unfortunately, science has sometimes been slow in accepting new ideas despite substantial evidence showing that the old paradigm is outdated and due for a change.

A brief historical account will suffice to indicate that this is true.

Scientists initially didn't believe in meteorites falling from the sky even though the phenomenon was repeatedly encountered by farmers. Ignaz Semmelweis was confined to a mental institution (where he sadly died at the age of forty-seven) for research that showed that death rates during childbirth plummeted if the doctors sanitized themselves before seeing their patients. Even the now commonly accepted idea of continental drift advocated by Alfred Wegener was rejected for decades because it was believed that if his hypothesis was accepted, many of the previous geological theories would have to be rewritten.[4]

Each of these ideas was considered heretical when it was first proposed, because the idea was antithetical to the conventional dogma of the time. Yet, time has proven that the ideas were right after all.

Today, science is again rejecting out of hand many phenomena such as 'extra-sensory perception' or sixth sense, the presence of spirits and the power of prayer.

The Basis for the Scientific Method Should Be Evidence, Not Theory

Reading all this, you may think that I am against science and the scientific method. Nothing is further from the truth. Science as we know it today has been hijacked. It is now an instrument of politics rather than of truth.

Science as we initially conceived it to be was based on the idea that we could get a glimpse of reality through observation, experimentation and evidence. Therefore, the experience of anomalous events like the presence of spirits should be seen as evidence of something that seems to be beyond our current understanding of science. Open-minded scientists would then explore these anomalies to gain a better understanding of how reality works.

But this is not what is happening. Instead, scientists are denying that these anomalies exist by calling people who are reporting them as deluded, dishonest or hallucinating. Even when they grudgingly acknowledge that these phenomena exist, they insist that there is a reasonable explanation for them that fits *their* theories of how things work, even if their theories no longer fit the evidence.

I'm not against the scientific method; what I am against is the thinking that considers theories more important than evidence.

Our Beliefs are Shaped by the Culture and the Times We are Born Into

Theories are ultimately about what we believe to be true. Our beliefs are developed over time, and are a byproduct of the culture we live in and the conditioning we are exposed to. Many of our beliefs are accepted at face value because the time and effort needed to make our own observations and tests to prove or disprove them is too onerous to make it viable.

For example, we have generally accepted that the Earth is round — although we ourselves have never seen the Earth from space. We believe in the idea of a round Earth based on the experience of Columbus and photos from space.

After all, when Columbus set sail from Spain at the end of the 15th century, everyone in Europe believed that the world was flat, and that Columbus was going to sail over the edge. Right?

Not quite. You see, even though that was the story we were taught in school and therefore what we accept as truth, the story is a myth.

By the end of the fourth century BC, Greeks already knew the Earth was round. That information had been passed (through writing) to anyone in Europe who had a basic education. People poured cold water on Columbus not because they thought the world was flat but because they believed that based on the technology of the day it would be impossible for a craft to travel west from Western Europe to the coasts of Asia. The distance involved was too far — and they were right.

What they didn't know then was that there were two undiscovered continents — the North and South American continents — that were between the two land masses of Asia and Europe.[5]

I mentioned the story of Columbus to prove a point: what we generally accept as truth is what authority figures, mainstream media and scientists tell us is true. Hence, we wrongly believe, based on what we were taught in school, that in Columbus's time people believed the world was flat.

Truth would be easy to distinguish if everyone agreed on the same facts based on what they saw, and opinions did not factor into the equation. This of course can never be true. Our version of history is shaped by which side we listen to; for example, the typical Japanese or North American citizen would have a very different opinion on the necessity of the atomic bombs dropped on Hiroshima and Nagasaki, Japan.

Similarly, our version of science and truth is shaped by the authorities — politicians, scientists, historians, etc — of the period in which we learn that version. In fact, much of what we now believe to be true was settled by debate and argument occurring long before we were born.

The Scientific Revolution Determined What We Should Believe

For example, it was not until the scientific revolution during the Age of Enlightenment in Europe in the 18th century that the authority figures of the time decided that rationality had to be the order of the day, in order to break from the past.

People who continued with their past traditions, who held on to ancient wisdoms, would become a threat to this 'new world order'. Therefore, a myth was created which has become our mainstream view of life: the myth of progress.

We believe today that our society is progressing, that we are smarter and more knowledgeable than our ancestors were solely on the basis that we live after them. As a result, past knowledge and wisdom have no value to modern society. This hidden belief is of course what permitted, if not encouraged, the later decimation and conversion of 'primitive' people — like the Native Americans of the US — based on our perceived superiority.

Before the Enlightenment, people believed there was a consciousness that could communicate with and through us; that the world was 'sacred' and that we were part of a wider web of life, that everything was interconnected.

With the 'new science', the universe is now thought to be just dead matter, without any consciousness to enliven it. If consciousness exists at all it was created by matter. Most importantly, for something to be real it has to be material.

Is Everything Real Necessarily Material?

The ironic thing is that no one has ever proven, or even tried to prove, that the statement that everything that is real has to be material is true. It was simply assumed by the founders of science. To this day, it is still assumed — believed true without proof — by scientists.

Anything that does not fit in with this assumption is therefore, by definition, false. Therefore, spirits aren't accepted as truth not because people don't experience them — they did before and they do today — but because spirits do not fit into the scientific model of the universe assumed by scientists. The logic is that since spirits *couldn't* possibly exist, they *didn't* exist.

Reasoned that way, it is easy to see how 'logical' science really is if it is based on theories and opinions shaped by a small group of people who want to maintain the status quo. Throw in a mixture of politics, power and authority into the brew and you start to see how a few people at the top, especially editors of prestigious scientific journals, can determine what is to be considered as truth for the majority of us who don't have the time, resources or interest to find out for ourselves.

That is why I mentioned previously that science as we now know it is not so much about truth but about politics and power.

The role of the powers-that-be in this situation is easy to find and assign blame to; there is however, another, more subtle process at work as well. This process is known as *cognitive dissonance*, and occurs in our mind.

Cognitive Dissonance Causes Us to Continue to Hold On to Our Beliefs despite Evidence to the Contrary

If something we observe or are exposed to fits in with our existing belief system, we feel comfortable in our worldview. If some information we see, hear or read doesn't agree with our existing beliefs (like some of the information in this book), we start to feel an internal conflict, a *dissonance*, within us. To relieve ourselves of this dissonance, the easiest way is to dismiss this new information.

Nicolai, whom we met in the Introduction (page 21), did not believe in the existence of ghosts even though he saw them himself because accepting that would have led to tremendous cognitive dissonance.

We create our reality through our beliefs. Anything that doesn't fit in with our beliefs becomes untrue for us. Therefore, the scientist who chooses to believe that everything that is real must necessarily be material will notice just the examples around him that prove his beliefs true.

Someone else who does believe in non-material phenomenon will also find that *her* reality will include the presence of these unseen forces.

If these two different groups of people meet, they argue endlessly from their own perspectives. It is a futile effort to expect a meeting of minds: whatever each group experiences, whatever is true for each, is a reflection of the beliefs they hold, and since their beliefs are different, they can never come to agreement.

Spontaneous Remissions and Placebo Effect as Anomalies in Allopathic Medicine

So how does this apply to medicine and health?

There are now many anomalies showing up in allopathic medicine, but the status quo remains strong because anyone who has dared to advocate that it was time to change the paradigm has been vilified, humiliated or threatened. Many of the pioneers I introduce throughout the book have done what they did at great personal risk to themselves, and their career was often curtailed because of what they did.

What are some examples of these anomalies in allopathic medicine?

We cover some of these in this chapter, but the entire book is about these anomalies. You will come to see that this book has been written because the anomalies viewed together tell a compelling story, a story that if understood would radically change the way we look at disease.

Spontaneous Remission

Let's look firstly at the little-known phenomenon of *spontaneous remission*, the medical term given for the unexpected, full and complete healing of a condition. It is considered unexpected when the person who had the spontaneous remission:

- Did not go for the treatment she was recommended to take;
- Underwent treatments which would not be considered sufficient for a cure; or
- Had a condition deemed medically incurable, ie there were no medical treatments available for that condition.

In one case, a child who was nearly one year old was suffering from a lung disease and treated without success by doctors. This form of lung disease was considered almost always fatal. Desperate, the family took him to a healing service at a church. Within five days, he showed signs of improvement. At a follow-up four years later, he was found to have completely recovered.[6]

The Institute of Noetic Sciences has documented at least 1,385 of these cases. Specifically, 1,051 of these involve spontaneous remission of cancer and 334 to spontaneous remission of other illnesses.[7]

It is easy to dismiss these as probable wrong diagnoses or due to 'unknown factors'. But 'unknown factors' just indicates that there is something that we do not know based on our current idea of how the world works. If these factors are known, these spontaneous remissions may not be considered anomalous at all.

We will cover what I believe are these unknown factors when I go into the model of how disease actually arises in Part II of the book.

Placebo Effect

Another anomaly is an unexplained (at least to conventional science) yet pervasive phenomenon called the *placebo effect*. In fact, it is so pervasive that in order for any new drug to be approved, its developers have to show that it can achieve results far superior to a placebo in a *double-blind study*.

A placebo is a medication made to be similar-looking to the drug being tested but without any active *pharmacological* ingredients, ie ingredients causing a physiological or biological reaction through drug action. In short, a placebo should theoretically have no effect on the person taking it.

Double-blind studies refer to studies where the patients are separated into two groups. One group of patients has the drug administered to it while the other group is given a placebo, but — and this is the important part — neither the medical personnel involved in administering the drug nor the patients involved in the study know which group is getting the drug and which the placebo.

The reason double-blind studies are considered the *gold standard* of drug trials is because it has been clearly shown that if the doctors or patients involved in a trial know which pill is the drug and which the placebo, their expectations influence the results of the experiments.[8]

Imagine a sugar pill taken as a placebo. This sugar pill, chemically *inert* (inactive) as far as providing any useful substances to the body, should not be at all effective, yet it has been shown that placebos like sugar pills can cure patients in about 35 percent of cases.[9]

It is often disparagingly claimed that the placebo is 'all in the mind'. But this has been proven to be untrue. Taking a placebo (when you don't know you are taking one) produces biological effects which can be physically observed. For example, a placebo was used to cure stomach ulcers around 33 percent to 38 percent of the time in clinical trials. When an endoscope was used to peer into the stomach, the ulcer was no longer physically present![10]

The biological effects when you take a placebo (thinking it's the real deal) have now been explained: they are the release of natural painkillers known as endorphins. When a group of scientists led by Jon Levine administered naloxone to a patient, they found that naloxone could reverse the pain-reducing effects of a placebo. Naloxone works by blocking the receptor sites in the brain usually reserved for endorphins. By blocking these sites, naloxone prevented the cells in the brain from taking up the endorphins released by the body when taking the placebo.[11]

Though we now have a physical explanation for the placebo effect, scientists are still perplexed. They have no theories to explain how simply *believing* — an act that belongs to the mental realm — that one is receiving help by taking a substance, whether the drug or the placebo, can possibly create a physical effect, in this case the release of endorphins in the body.

The placebo effect should not happen, according to our conventional understanding of physics and chemistry. If the mind can indeed influence the body, many theories about how health and disease work would have to be revised. The placebo response indicates that a patient's beliefs, expectations, desires and hopes can play an integral part in the healing process.[12] This is something that mainstream scientists are still vehemently denying.

In a kind of perverse way, mainstream scientists like to use the placebo effect to explain away the effects of all *complementary therapies*, ie any therapies that are not part of the allopathic model of drugs and surgery, because that is the easiest way to dismiss any and all anomalies without needing to understand them.

However, placebo effects, though present, cannot be the sole mechanism by which complementary therapies obtain healing results. There are cases of healing in people who were not even aware that they were being worked on by healers, a phenomenon known as *remote healing*. [13] There are also cases of healing results demonstrated on animals like rats whose very nature means that they cannot be subjected to the placebo effect (which requires a human being to believe, this being a higher, cognitive, thought process that is not believed to be available to animals). [14]

Summary

Science has advanced whenever we have had a new understanding about how things work. Anomalies, or exceptions to the rule, point the way to these new paradigms and perspectives.

Unfortunately, science tends to stick to the conventional. Changes in the scientific field thus tend to take a long time to come. One reason for this has to do with cognitive dissonance. We tend to accept ideas based on what we currently believe, and these beliefs are shaped by the culture and times we are born in.

So for scientists who have been trained in a certain way of thinking — that things that are real are necessarily material, a thinking perpetuated by the Scientific Revolution of the 1700s — it is hard to accept the anomalies that are surfacing.

This phenomenon is also happening in medicine. For example, we see that spontaneous remissions and placebo effects are two anomalies in medicine that suggest that our understanding of health and disease is not complete.

Science as we know it is no longer just about evidence; it is also about opinions and power. As we shall see in the next chapter, this is also playing out in medicine.

This would have been fine if the allopathic medicine model had continued to serve the people who came to it and was effective in curing disease. But let's see how it is actually performing.

TWO — Medicine: How We May Be Getting Sicker, Not Healthier

Cures for Cancer Are Currently Suppressed

Royal Raymond Rife may have found the cure for cancer. Yet, instead of being awarded a Nobel Prize for it, he lost his laboratory, and information about his work is still suppressed. To understand why, we have to look at who Rife, as he was known by his peers, was.

Rife was born in 1888 in Nebraska, USA. After medical school he went on to work in the Carl Zeiss Optical Company in Germany. Based on the knowledge of optical lenses he gained there, he invented the Universal Microscope, which was able to see the tiniest *microorganisms* (bacteria, fungi, mold and viruses) in the blood and tissues.

Using the Universal Microscope, he realized that 1) every microorganism had its own particular electro-magnetic frequency, and 2) cancer was linked to a previously unknown micro-organism he called BX. Rife discovered he could use specific frequencies to kill bacteria or viruses in the human body without causing damage to the surrounding tissue.

Based on his research, Rife developed the Rife machine, a device that generated a variable frequency. The device could be tuned to produce a frequency that matched the oscillatory rate of a bacterium or virus, making the microorganism implode and effectively destroying it without disturbing normal cells. This effect is based on *resonance*. An example of resonance you may be familiar with is using a high-pitched sound of a particular frequency to shatter glass.

In 1934, in a trial conducted at the University of Southern California (USC), he was presented with 16 terminally ill patients suffering from different kinds of cancer. After three months of treatment using his Rife machine, fourteen of these patients fully recovered; after a further three months, the remaining two also recovered. This was a 100 percent recovery rate — and that too in only six months!

One body that took strong interest in the Rife machine was the American Medical Association (AMA). (The AMA is supposed to be an independent trade organization for doctors, but pharmaceutical companies played a leading role in the establishment and funding of this organization.) Not only had the machine succeeded where the pharmaceutical companies had failed but it did not require expensive surgery or drugs.

If the Rife machine were to become the standard treatment for cancer, it would seriously undermine the financial positions of the pharmaceutical companies. When the AMA's attempt to buy over the rights to produce the Rife machines was refused, a series of events happened.

First Rife was branded a quack by AMA; anyone associated with him was told to stop the association or risk losing his medical license.

Then his laboratory was mysteriously burnt down one night.

Finally, one of his greatest supporters, Dr. Milbank Johnson, died of suspicious circumstances ('poisoned' was the term coined by federal inspectors). The documents of the USC medical trials of the 16 cancer patients disappeared at the same time.

Rife died a broken man in 1970.[15]

You may think this incident with Rife is an isolated incident.

Unfortunately, it's not. Many effective Complementary and Alternative Medicine (CAM) treatments for cancer currently exist, but you will not hear about them for the simple fact that information on these treatments is being suppressed. The only options offered by allopathic medicine for cancer are chemotherapy, radiotherapy (radiation therapy) and surgery.

I know it's difficult to believe that the US medical system would deliberately suppress a treatment that can help so many suffering people. The plain reason is that the modern medical system prioritizes profit over the welfare of the people it purportedly is helping.

What I'm talking about here is the system, not the people involved. In fact, I believe the majority of medical professionals chose the medical professions to make a difference in the life of the suffering and the sick. They had hoped through their efforts to eradicate disease, alleviate pain and suffering, and create a world of healthy people.

So what happened? To answer this question, we need to look at a brief history of medicine.

Our Current Allopathic Medical System is Based on Politics and Money

Western medicine can be traced to ancient Egypt and Greece.

Hippocrates, the father of Western medicine, was Greek. He was the first to propose that disease should be linked to natural, external and not supernatural, causes. (On that score, he wasn't right, but I am jumping ahead of myself. In Chapter Eleven I speak about the link between disease and spirits.)

Hippocrates believed in a vital force that animated the body; he also did not believe in strong intervention to bring the body back to balance. Contrast this with another school of thought — the School of Cnidos — which believed in first relieving the symptoms of the illness.

Both schools existed side by side until the mid-1800s when the Cnidian School prevailed because it was in line with the material sciences of the period.

Nicolai, whom we met in the Introduction (page 21), received a treatment protocol known as bloodletting. This was devised by another great physician of ancient Greece, Galen, who taught that illness resulted from an imbalance in the various 'humors' of the body, things like bile and blood.

Medical students at the time were taught to remedy this imbalance by uncomfortable practices like purging and bloodletting. Paracelsus, a Swiss-German physician, was a strong opponent of Galen's philosophy: he advocated the use of herbs and plants instead of violent bloodletting. Being one of the first to recommend chemical cures for afflictions, he set the stage for the pharmaceuticals we have today.

In the centuries that followed, technological advances such as the microscope began to shift the focus of attention to the external causes of disease. By the beginning of the nineteenth century, two major schools of thought had developed. The allopaths believed in strong intervention against disease, using toxic chemicals to treat the symptoms. The homeopaths, on the other hand, believed in the natural recuperative powers of the body and utilized special preparations based mainly on plant extracts.

Then the wealthy people of that time, people like the Rockefellers, came up with a brilliant business idea that would transform medicine forever.

They would finance the allopathic cause by creating a health system based on the prescription of drugs for which they would have a virtual monopoly, and prevent others from sticking their hands in this same pie. The AMA was their vehicle to accomplish this. Note that the AMA is not a government organization but a privately-run organization similar to trade unions.[16]

The American Medical Association (AMA) Takes Over the Health Industry

In 1906, the Council on Medical Education, an AMA body founded to 'improve medical education in the US', started cracking down on schools that did not teach its way of practicing medicine, ie treatments based predominantly on drugs.

A scientific research methodology —, which evolved to become the 'randomized, double-blind, placebo-controlled' study, considered the gold standard of drug studies — popular in German universities was brought to the US by Abraham Flexner. In 1910, the Flexner Report was issued; it provided funding only to schools, research institutions and other associated bodies that followed this methodology. Funding to institutions that followed other methodologies was barred.

Then in 1913, a Propaganda Department (real name!) was set up to change people's opinions of what was considered proper medicine and what was to be known as 'fraud' and 'quackery'.

In one fell swoop, anything that did not meet the approving eyes of the AMA became subject to attacks: ancient traditional medicine, homeopathy, chiropractic, and a host of others. Folk medicines were branded as superstition and trivialized. All therapies that did not utilize pharmaceutical medicines become known as alternative medicines, ie alternative to allopathic medicine. The irony is that AMA, which was created only in 1847, was denouncing other medical approaches such as Traditional Chinese Medicine (TCM), which has been around for over 2,000 years.[17]

How Scientific and Effective are Modern Medicine, Really?

It's commonly believed that pharmaceutical drugs in the allopathic model go through a rigorous process from which only the safest and most effective drugs are approved for use.

But the truth is that up to 75 percent of all the published research on pharmaceutical drugs in prestigious journals like the Journal of American Medical Association (JAMA) is authored by public relations firms hired by pharmaceutical companies. This research routinely understates the dangerous side-effects of the drugs.[18]

This has led to a number of notorious drug recalls: Vioxx in 2004, recalled for increased risk of heart attacks and strokes; Baycol in 2001, after more than 100,000 deaths had been attributed to this drug for high-cholesterol; and Fen-Phen in 1997, after patients wanting to lose weight also developed increased heart problems.[19]

How about how allopathic medicine has actually performed? In 2004, Gary Null, Ph.D., a nutritionist, and a group of other researchers showed that if all the annual deaths — both inpatient and outpatient — in the United States were categorized by cause of death, medicine would actually be the number 1 killer, outranking even heart disease and cancer! This includes errors from prescribing the wrong medication, and fatal, adverse drug reactions, which can happen even when a drug is properly given and administered.[20]

Also shocking is how ineffective drugs really are. Dr. Allen Roses, a vice president at GlaxoSmithKline, said in 2003 that more than 90 percent of all drugs work only in 30-50 percent of the patients taking them.[21]

Of course, our current medical system is not without its strengths. For traumas and emergencies (eg, severe pain, accidents, etc), no one thinks twice about receiving care in hospitals; there is definitely a place for surgery in life-threatening conditions. Yet, in the case of *chronic* illnesses (illnesses that persist a long time or constantly recur) like depression, chronic fatigue and multiple sclerosis, many patients struggle despite the best medical care and drugs medicine has to offer.

The reason is simple: allopathic medicine has a distinct set of beliefs and philosophies that sometimes runs counter to what is truly beneficial for the body.

Anti-Inflammatory Drugs May Do More Harm than Good in the Long-Term

For example, let's look at the preoccupation in allopathic medicine with anti-inflammatory drugs.

At first sight, the logic is impeccable. Inflammation, which is characterized by swelling and fatigue, creates pain and can limit mobility. Taking anti-inflammatory drugs to relieve pain makes going about one's daily life much easier.

However, even as far back as 1952, the famous theory of *homotoxicology*, developed by Dr. Hans-Heinrich Reckweg of Germany, had thrown into disarray the idea that anti-inflammatory drugs are necessarily good for us.[22] Let's see why.

Dr. Hans-Heinrich believed that the body has a natural state of balance known as *homeostasis*. For example, our body maintains our internal temperature at around 37 degrees Celsius; we have an 'internal thermostat' that works to cool us down through perspiration if we get heated to over that temperature, and an involuntary shivering mechanism to raise our internal temperature if we fall below that critical level.

Toxins are influences that disturb our natural state. For example, exposure to pesticides — substances foreign to the body — can lead to hormonal changes in the body that move us away from our natural state. Pesticides are therefore considered toxic to the human body.

The main ways to remove unwanted substances and toxins from the body include perspiration through the skin, excretion through the colon, and elimination through the liver and kidneys. In a healthy person, elimination happens automatically and the body is able to remove all the toxins in the body. However, if elimination becomes compromised for any reason, the body goes into the inflammatory response phase.

Inflammation allows the body to heal the injury while preventing the toxin from doing further damage. Colds, fever, pimples, vomiting, diarrhea: all these are attempts by the body to push out toxins. Only when the toxins are eliminated to the body's satisfaction does the inflammation clear up.

For instance, let's look at why fever, a form of inflammatory response, can be helpful. Fever causes our immune cells to divide more quickly while slowing down the proliferation of bacteria that love dampness and cold. As the increase in body temperature requires the body to expend more energy than usual (approximately 10 percent more energy for every one degree Celsius rise), the brain compensates by generating feelings of lethargy so that excess energy can be diverted to fighting the infection.[23]

If this natural process of inflammation is not allowed to complete — for example through the administration of *antipyretics* (drugs that reduce fever) — the toxins may get pushed deeper into the body. In experiments where sick animals are treated with antipyretics, the animals are more likely to die from infection than recover from illness.[24]

As more and more toxins enter the body over time, some of these toxins became encased in the structure of our body. This weakens our bones, tissues and organs over time, and may cause the body to utilize backup systems to compensate. For example, if the liver and the kidneys become overwhelmed dealing with detoxification, they may push the toxins out through the skin, creating psoriasis or eczema. Alternatively, sinus problems may develop if the mucous membranes are utilized as a back-up for detoxification. The body can also store all these toxins in growths, whether internally as fibroids and tumors (which may eventually turn cancerous) or externally as warts and cysts.

All these backup systems are not meant to last forever, or even for a long time. The body is meant to eliminate the stored toxins so it can return to homeostasis.

But every time we take more anti-inflammatories to stop the inflammation the body produces to kick-start elimination of a toxin, we effectively begin a 'civil war' within our body! Seen in that light the logic of anti-inflammatories doesn't look so strong after all.

Each time a healing process is disrupted, the body gets weaker and healing time lengthens. Inflammation symptoms like pain and fatigue get progressively worse. If the body is unable to rid itself of toxins, these 'poisons' start to affect the stomach and liver before gradually affecting more delicate organs such as the kidneys and lungs. Finally, the disease will reach the brain and heart, our most critical organs. When our vital energies get fully exhausted, the body collapses. Eventually death ensues.

In summary then, the progression of disease goes through six stages. A later stage is initiated only when the previous stage can no longer bring the body back to balance.

The first stage is *elimination* of toxins through pimples, coughing, diarrhea and vomiting when normal elimination processes like moving your bowels, urination and perspiration are insufficient.

In the second stage of *inflammation*, the body isolates the toxins by producing a swelling around the injured area and making the person feel tired so that resting and healing can take place.

In the third stage, *deposition*, the body creates storage sites — such as fibroids, warts, gout and kidney stones — to store the waste products that are not eliminated quickly enough.

The next three stages are *impregnation*, where waste products are incorporated into bodily tissues when they cannot be eliminated;

degeneration, or rapid death of cells, possibly leading to organ failure; and *dedifferentiation*, where the body has given up and has actively begun a process of disintegration.

Interestingly, Dr. Hans-Heinrich noticed that in the early stages of disease, the reactions tend to center round the 'humors' of yore: blood, lymph, phlegm and bile. That would explain why bloodletting and purging, the dominant ways of treatment during the 18th and 19th centuries, could effect improvements in the body. They might have permitted toxins to be eliminated through these unorthodox methods.

Of course, in no way am I advocating these practices in modern times: it is now possible to eliminate these toxins in less invasive ways. The point is that the medieval physicians who used bloodletting and purging as therapeutic practices in the past may have known a thing or two after all. They were not, necessarily, merely the ignorant quacks that our modern society has made them out to be.

Our Body is Not Just a Machine with Separate Parts

Another flaw in allopathic medicine is its preference for treating the body as a machine, and reducing the body to its different components and parts, instead of viewing it as a whole system that is interconnected. We have specialists for the digestive system, specialists for the heart, and specialists for the brains, amongst many others. Yet these organs do not work in isolation.

For example, recent evidence indicates a strong link between our mental well-being and the health of the gut. Mice born by *Caesarean* birth (also known as a *C-section*, in which incisions are made in the mother's abdomen to facilitate delivery), leading to a very different bacterial environment in the gut as compared to mice born naturally, were found to be significantly more depressed and anxious. This of course also has implications for babies born through C-section. By not getting the chance to pick up bacteria from the mother's vagina during birth, these babies are more susceptible to mental illnesses later on in life.[25]

The claim that one organ (the gut) can influence another organ (the brain) was made by holistic practitioners a long time ago, but was met with withering skepticism by neuroscientists. Part of this resistance occurs because neuroscientists have been trained to isolate our mental state to the brain. Just like a person who wields only a hammer starts to see every problem as a nail, people who specialize in the brain tend to see all problems as originating from the brain. Introducing the gut into the equation is thus a profane idea, at least from the neuroscientists' perspective.

Summary

The reason the US's allopathic medical system is the way it is can actually be traced to the setting up of the AMA and how it took over the healthcare system. There are certain materialist paradigms — the body is purely physical, inflammation is bad and should be suppressed, the body is a machine with parts that can be separated instead of being seen as a holistic whole — which cause medicine to be much less effective than it should be.

I am NOT advocating 'Either-or', as in EITHER allopathic medicine OR complementary medicine. I AM advocating 'And': both allopathic medicine and complementary medicine. Both should be acknowledged as useful, with the approach to take depending on the context and the situation that the patient finds herself in.

It is generally acknowledged that complementary medicine is good for the prevention of disease, and for helping to alleviate chronic illnesses or conditions.

Allopathic medicine comes into its own when disease has progressed to the point that surgery or life-saving drugs are likely to be the only options left.

In the next chapter, I discuss another core principle of allopathic medicine: that the body is purely material, in stark contrast to the view of complementary medicine that the body is intimately tied to consciousness.

THREE — Consciousness: Shaper of the Physical Body

Near-Death Experiences Suggest Consciousness Survives Beyond the Death of the Body

Pam Reynolds Lowery was in mortal trouble. Her scan showed a large aneurysm that was so close to the brain stem that that her chances of survival were deemed virtually zero.

Her neurosurgeon, Dr. Robert F. Spetzler, proposed, as a final desperate measure, a radical surgery known as a *standstill operation* in which Pam's body temperature would be lowered to 10 degrees Celsius, blood would be drained from her head and all breathing and heartbeats would cease.

Pam was clinically dead — defined as having no measurable brain wave activity — during the entire surgery that lasted around 7 hours.

The operation was a total success and Pam eventually recovered fully. She had the operation when she was 35, and went on to live to the age of 53 years.

The operation sounds like a medical miracle, but the real miracle happened when Pam was revived. She was able to describe accurately medical equipment that was not in the operating room when she was awake but that was later used in the operation. She could also accurately describe a conversation that took place in the operating room while she was being operated on.

When asked how she was aware of all this information, she said that right after she went under anesthesia, she found herself above the operating room looking down at her body and all the medical personnel performing the operation. At one point, she felt herself being pulled towards a light. In the light, she could see her grandmother, an uncle and other relatives who had passed on. She had felt better in that light then she had ever felt in body, and had not wanted to return to her body until her uncle pushed her back.[26]

Pam's experience is known as a Near-Death Experience (NDE), and it is not as rare as we think. Dr. Pim van Lommel, a cardiologist in the Netherlands, interviewed around 344 survivors of heart failure in 1988. He found that 18 percent of them reported recollection and memories after clinical death. Several of the survivors independently reported events such as moving through a tunnel, meeting dead relatives, or experiencing a review of their life. In some cases, a blind patient was even able to 'see' and describe what she saw during the NDE experience![27]

This goes against all conventional medical thinking: the brain is supposed to be the physical *substrate* (layer) for the mind. Once the brain dies, the mind should also die — so the dogma goes.

However, there seems to be a consciousness that continues even after death, suggesting that some part of our mind is not purely physical, and does not depend on the brain for its awareness.

Allopathic Medicine Splits Up Mind and Body

This split between the mind and the body has been at the forefront of conflicts between people who believe in a universe that is purely mechanical and physical, and those who believe that the universe comprises not just physical substances but also an intangible, non-physical component that is the basis of our consciousness.

This conflict is especially pronounced in medicine. The basis of allopathic medicine is that since the body is only physical, all effective healing must have a purely physical basis and anything that smacks of 'energy healing' is highly suspect. For example, if there is a tumor, surgery is the only option. Since the mind and the body are separate, nothing that is of the mind — thoughts, emotions or consciousness — should have an impact on the physical body.

But there is a growing number of people advocating the idea that consciousness creates our material reality instead of the other way around, based on evidence gathered from research in fields as diverse as quantum physics (the science of the smallest particles) and *psychoneuroimmunology* (the study of how thoughts and emotions influence the nervous and immune system).

Consciousness Influences the Material World, As Demonstrated in the Double-Slit Experiment

We see how consciousness influences the material world in the famous double-slit experiment conducted by Thomas Young in 1801. At this time, there was fierce debate on whether light was a wave or a particle.

In Young's experiment (see figure next page), a light was shone in front of a screen that had two holes placed very close together. The resulting image was then projected onto a second screen. When the distance between the holes in the first screen was made smaller and smaller, Young started seeing light and dark lines, which indicated interference patterns consistent with the fact that light was made up of waves. Thanks in large part to this experiment, the consensus throughout the nineteenth century was that light behaved like a wave.

Then, 104 years later in March 1905, Albert Einstein formulated the *quantum theory of light*: the idea that light exists as tiny, fixed packets, or particles, of energy that he called photons.

How could light be both wave and particle at the same time?

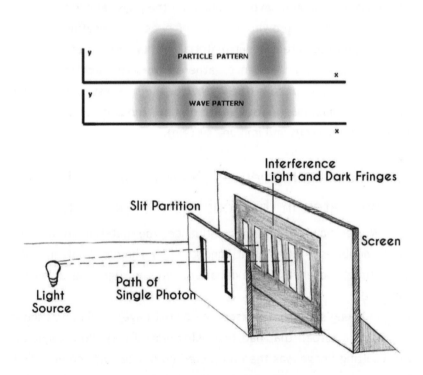

Figure 2: Young's Double-Slit Experiment

Light *does* seem to have features of both waves and particles; whether it acts as a wave or as a particle depends on whether it is being observed!

In the double-slit experiment, when the photon detectors used to track the path of the light beam were switched on, the photons were seen to travel through only one slit at a time. This meant light acted as a particle when observed by the detector. The moment the photon detectors were switched off, the wave interference pattern returned, indicating that light was now acting as a wave.[28]

A scientist called Dean Radin performed an extension of the double-slit experiment. Experienced meditators were placed in a room separate from the experiment, and asked to place their awareness on the light beam. No photon detectors were used; the meditators would function as 'human photon detectors'. After nine rounds of remote observation, they found that the results of using the meditators as 'observers' were similar to those when using the photon detectors in Young's experiment. Light behaved like a particle when the meditators were viewing it remotely, and like a wave when they were not observing it.[29]

The only possible explanation for this is that observation changes our physical reality. In other words, we cannot observe something without simultaneously changing it. Most remarkable of all, as shown by the experiment with the meditators, this observation is not limited by space or distance. Simply imagining being there, observing the phenomenon, seems to give the same results at the quantum level as being physically there!

Extra-Sensory Perception and Effects on Random Number Generators Suggest That Consciousness Does Influence the Material World

Two other examples further demonstrate that consciousness does have a profound impact on material reality.

The first example is a phenomenon observed when testing for Extra-Sensory Perception (ESP). ESP has always been a controversial topic; sceptics claim that any perception outside of our normal five senses is impossible.

It has been observed before that in tests to verify ESP, believers of ESP tended to do better than non-believers. This effect has become known as the 'sheep-goat effect', sheep representing the believers and goats being the disbelievers.

A psychologist called Tony Lawrence, who was then studying this phenomenon as a graduate student, surveyed over 685,000 guesses by 4,500 participants over a period of 50 years between 1943 and 1993 (the year the research ended). He found that the sheep outperformed the goats in ESP tests by a margin so enormous that the odds of chance being able to explain this huge disparity were more than a trillion to one.[30]

In other words, if I believe in ESP, I tend to be more 'psychic' during ESP tests. Being a non-believer is a self-fulfilling prophecy: if I don't believe in ESP, I don't do well in the tests, and I therefore become even more convinced that ESP is a figment of people's imagination.

The second example is known as the Global Consciousness Project and deals with what we call *Random Number Generators*

(RNGs). These are machines hooked up to computers that are programmed to produce totally random numbers.

Imagine an experiment in which a friend throws a coin into the air. Over a huge number of throws, you should get heads or tails about 50 percent of the time, based purely on chance. Now imagine that you have to somehow 'influence the coin' to come up with many more heads than can be explained away statistically. If you do get heads and tails in about equal amounts, we can conclude that your consciousness was not able to influence the coin throw. Indeed, this is what we would expect in a purely material world.

However, researchers have discovered that when a large number of people, perhaps all over the world, are focusing on the same event — eg, the September 11 terrorist acts in the US, the Olympic Games every four years, and the death of Princess Diana in 1997 — RNGs running during the period begin generating non-random numbers. Indeed, this is exactly what was observed during the three events mentioned above. Hundreds of major events have been analyzed; researchers have found a significant correlation between the occurrence of such events and significant deviations from randomness in the numbers produced by RNGs operating in that period.

The conclusions seem clear: consciousness, especially mass consciousness, can have an impact on 'objective' outcomes.[31]

A corollary is that what we consider as objective research may not be so objective after all. The fundamental assumptions of scientific research — that there is an objective reality that is not shaped by our consciousness — may have to be revised!

If Consciousness Affects Physical Reality, Any Model Explaining Health and Diseases Has to Factor in Consciousness

Cell biologist Robert Lanza, famous for his stem-cell discoveries, came up with the concept of *biocentrism* that essentially states the same thing: consciousness creates reality instead of reality 'creating' observers like us.[32]

Sperry Andrews, who created the Human Connection Project, has found more than five hundred different scientific studies that prove that human consciousness can affect other life forms. I believe that the reason this is possible is that consciousness is present in every living thing. Consciousness can even influence inanimate systems like machines.[33] If this is true, it has important implications for healing.

Let's use a metaphor to illustrate this. Let's imagine that consciousness is the computer program, and the physical body is the printout from the computer program. An error with the printout — for instance, a spelling error — is equivalent to a problem in the physical body.

To fix this error in the print-out, we can use a liquid correction pen to erase the misspelling and then enter the new correct version. With our body, this is the equivalent of physical intervention like surgery. But if the computer program has a *bug* (software error) that keeps misspelling words, we have to keep using the liquid correction pen to fix the errors. Instead, the logical thing to do is go directly to the computer program to fix the bug so that we can resolve this issue of misspelling, at the source, once and for all.

3 - Consciousness: Shaper of the Physical Body

If our consciousness is what creates our material reality, including our body, then trying to resolve problems (disease) with the body via physical means can never be a permanent fix. We may actually be barking up the wrong tree by creating revolutionary new drugs and innovative surgical methods. No matter how much money we pump into research, we are essentially still looking at the print-out (a problem in the body) instead of the program that creates the print-out (the consciousness that creates the problem in the body).

All this reminds me of a Sufi story I once heard.

A neighbor found Nasruddin looking for something underneath a street lamp. When asked what he was searching for, Nasruddin replied that he was looking for his keys. The helpful neighbor started searching with him. After half an hour of effort, the two of them still couldn't find the keys. The neighbor asked Nasruddin to try to recall where he'd dropped the keys. Nasruddin pointed to another, dark corner of the street. Aghast, the neighbor asked him why he had been looking beneath the street lamp if the keys had not been dropped there in the first place. Nasruddin calmly replied "There is more light underneath the lamp, of course".[34]

Could we unknowingly be searching for the 'key of disease' where it's brightest and most obvious — the physical body — instead of where it can actually be found: in our consciousness?

Summary

Science splits up mind and body and considers them separate. Based on this principle, mind does not influence the body and since the body is physical, any medical intervention has to be necessarily physical.

Near-death experiences however suggest that the mind is not limited to the physical body and seems to survive beyond death. Other research like the double-slit experiment, extra-sensory perception studies, and effects of major, world-focusing events on random number generators strongly suggests that reality is shaped by consciousness.

If consciousness does have material effects, including effects on the physical body, then any model explaining health and disease has to factor in consciousness. Unfortunately, allopathic medicine is currently ignoring the problem of consciousness. As a result, it can never find Nasruddin's keys — the true keys to the cause of disease.

In Part II, I am going to describe my model of why and how diseases are caused. A person is a being of three parts: body, mind and soul. The concept of consciousness, as you will see, is very much linked to our soul, and plays a pivotal role in the model. Let's begin!

PART II
CRACKING THE
DISEASE CODE –
THE MODEL

FOUR — Stress: All Diseases are linked to Stress

Autism is connected to the Leaky Gut Syndrome

"We suspect Jay has autism. Unfortunately there is no cure for autism. This is a lifelong condition for him." With those words, Fiona's life would be changed forever.

Jay was Fiona's three-year-old son. Everything was fine until Jay was around 18 months old. He had been able to speak a few words, show good eye contact and get along well with everyone.

Then he started regressing. The few words he said could no longer be heard; he started screaming for no reason; and he no longer responded to his name being called.

In Singapore, where Jay lived, no confirmed diagnosis of autism is possible until the child is at least three years old. When Jay reached that age, Fiona brought him to see a pediatrician and her worse fears were confirmed.

In the months following, Fiona became a mother on a mission: she devoured the content of every website on autism she found. A constant theme ran through the information she read: many parents advocated putting the child on a gluten-free casein-free (GFCF) diet. Gluten is a protein found in wheat, and casein a protein found in milk.

Fiona went back to the pediatrician for advice.

"Oh, there is no scientific evidence to prove that the GFCF diet helps autistic children."

Undeterred, Fiona put Jay on a strict GFCF diet. Around one month into the protocol, Jay started responding. The screaming spells reduced, his eye contact improved, and he started speaking a few words again. The correlation between eliminating these two foods from Jay's diet, and the significant improvement in his condition, was clear. But why should this be happening?

All autistic children seem to suffer from a condition called *leaky gut syndrome*. (We had mentioned a link between mental health and the gut in Chapter Two, page 51. This link is also true for autism. What medical dogma considers a neurological and brain issue is instead closely connected to the gut.)

Leaky gut syndrome is a condition in which the gut's lining has become porous. The increased permeability of the gut allows undigested foods to pass through the intestinal barrier into the blood stream. The body, however, doesn't like any foreign substances in the blood stream. It flags these particles as harmful, and provokes an inflammatory response or allergic reaction.

Gluten and casein are proteins that don't get digested easily. (There are many reasons for this; most have to do with the way our modern, industrial, farming system currently processes wheat and milk.) These two proteins therefore are likelier than other food substances to produce an inflammatory reaction. With repeated inflammatory response, the immune system ends up attacking not just the particles in the blood stream but also other parts of the body, resulting in what are termed *autoimmune* conditions.

The immunity-system cells of the body are supposed to distinguish between what is 'self' and what is 'others'. To maintain the integrity of the body, foreign substances, especially those deemed to be harmful to the body, are neutralized by these immune cells. An *autoimmune condition* is a situation where the immune cells attack not just harmful organisms but also the cells of its own body.

Diseases considered autoimmune in nature include balding, rheumatoid arthritis and Hashimoto's Thyroiditis; there is a whole host of others. In fact, my hypothesis is that eventually we will discover that all illnesses are autoimmune in nature and originate from the gut. Thousands of years ago, Hippocrates, the father of modern medicine, made a statement that is now famous: "All disease begins in the gut."[35]

Alcoholism is connected to Adrenal Fatigue

Lena had been struggling with alcoholism for over ten years. She had been in and out of rehabilitation centers; every time she resolved to stop drinking, she would spiral into a depression and would end up drinking again. Her mother had also been an alcoholic; mother and daughter were considered the 'black sheep' of the family.

Lena's issue had a lot to do with a condition known as *adrenal fatigue* (although she wasn't initially aware of it). In order to boost her flagging energy, she was unconsciously self-medicating herself through stimulants. (Other stimulants besides alcohol include coffee, tea, sugar, gambling, sex, exercise, high-risk activities and hard drugs.) The purpose of these stimulants is to artificially prop up the adrenals. Unfortunately, the dosage required to maintain arousal intensities tend to increase over time. Since the boost is temporary, the adrenals eventually succumb to exhaustion. This explains why alcoholics start with a few drinks but over time need more and more to stay afloat. Before they realize it they are already deep in the throes of alcoholism.[36]

Anxiety is related to Thyroid Problems

Our final example is Eva who was experiencing anxiety and panic attacks, insomnia and muscle weaknesses.

Presented with these symptoms, an allopathic doctor tested Eva for her thyroid levels but the blood test results were in the normal range. She was given some sleeping pills and referred to a psychiatrist who put her on some anti-depressants to see how she would respond to them. Her symptoms didn't abate.

As she desperately searched for a solution by going to various doctors and specialists, they started to see her symptoms as of *psychosomatic* origin, ie her illness was just 'in her head'. That's how Eva finally turned to alternative therapies.

Eva's case is typical of many people with chronic illnesses. She had undiagnosed thyroid problems; laboratory tests uncover only a very small fraction of cases of people who are *hypothyroid* ('hypo' means low, so hypothyroids are people with low thyroid function). In fact, the Vascular Research Foundation in New York found that for over forty years, 85 percent of their patients who had passed the standard tests — indicating that they had normal thyroid function — had nevertheless demonstrated an improvement in their condition with thyroid supplementation.[37]

The thyroid gland, located in the neck, is responsible for releasing hormones that control growth, body metabolism, energy levels, temperature and mood. The thyroid hormone serves a critical function in the body. Space does not permit me to list down all the benefits of having the right amount of thyroid hormones in the body. Let me mention just three examples of the serious problems that can occur when your thyroid function is sub-optimal. I am sure you will recognize people around you who have these problems.

Firstly, the thyroid controls body temperature and can therefore affect brain function. If the temperature of the body is lowered, there are changes in brain wave patterns. This can cause deterioration in brain response and processing, mental activity, memory, response, or motor co-ordination, or lead to all kinds of sensory issues. [38] Children who have developmental delays – eg, autism, ADHD, Down's syndrome – probably have thyroids acting sub-optimally.

Secondly, thyroid hormone balance is vital for mood. If the thyroid is overactive *(hyperthyroidism)*, the person slips easily into anxiety and panic; conversely, if the thyroid is underactive *(hypothyroidism)*, symptoms like depression and fatigue develop. [39] Anyone suffering from mental illnesses – from suicidal tendencies to schizophrenia – can probably trace the condition to their thyroid function.

Thirdly, low thyroid function also affects metabolism and weight. [40] So anyone who is obese or struggling with weight issues probably has a thyroid problem. This explains why many people diet and exercise religiously without making a dent in their weight.

The Biochemistry of Stress Is Activated Through the HPA Axis

To understand how all these conditions are linked to stress, let's review the biochemistry of stress.

The stress response is coordinated by our *endocrine organs*, particularly the hypothalamus, pituitary gland and adrenals, known as the *HPA Axis* (see Figure 4: Effects of Stress on the Body on page 76). After the nervous system, the endocrine system is the second system of intercellular communication in the body. It is a collection of glands that secrete hormones directly into the bloodstream.

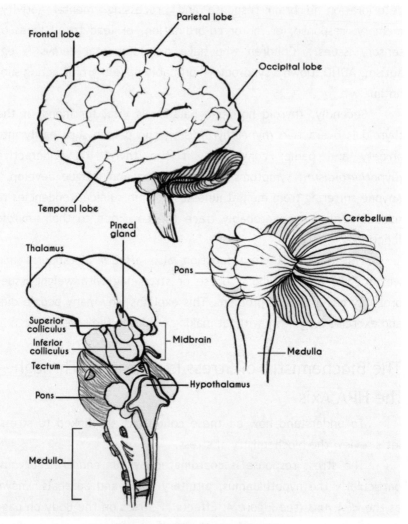

Figure 3: The Human Brain

The hypothalamus (see figure on previous page), which is part of the brain, regulates vital bodily functions such as hunger, thirst, fluid concentrations, body temperature, reproductive processes, emotional states, aggressive behaviors and response to stress. It works closely with the pituitary gland, which is also known as the 'master gland' (though that's wrong — it's really the hypothalamus that's the master gland) for its ability to release hormones that stimulate and regulate other glands. The adrenal glands sit just above the kidneys, and secrete cortisol and other hormones during emergencies.

When a person experiences stress, the hypothalamus releases a hormone (called CRH) that stimulates the pituitary gland to release another hormone (called ACTH) which acts on the adrenal cortex. The adrenal glands secrete *steroid hormones* (cortisol, adrenaline and noradrenaline), with the most prominent being cortisol. [41] In fact, as we shall see, cortisol's role in the whole equation of disease is pivotal.

Cortisol Plays a Key Role in Disease by Causing the Conditions of Leaky Gut Syndrome, Adrenal Fatigue and Hypothyroidism / Hyperthyroidism

Let's first examine how cortisol causes leaky gut syndrome, adrenal fatigue and thyroid dysfunction.

Under normal circumstances, cortisol regulates the immune system. To understand how important the immune system is, recall what happens if you cut yourself with a knife while cutting the vegetables. The blood clots automatically; in less than a week, you have at most a minor scar to show for the accident.

The immune system has a marvelous ability to self-heal. In fact, all medical devices, drugs, surgical interventions, conventional therapies or complementary therapies merely support this innate ability of the immune system. Ultimately, the only thing that can heal the body is your own immune system. Research from Stanford University Medical School shows that cells that are open and in growth / healing mode — a fully functioning immune system — are literally immune to illness and disease![42]

During stress however, the cortisol level become elevated. An elevated cortisol level means that a particular substance known as SIgA that helps regenerate the gut lining is slow in being produced. In the long term, this leads to the laceration of the gut lining, leading to the leaky gut syndrome.[43]

Since 80 percent of our immune system is found in the gut, the leaky gut syndrome causes the immune function to become suppressed.[44]

When the immune system can no longer adequately defend against *pathogenic* (disease-causing) microbes such as harmful bacteria, parasites and yeast, we get an overgrowth of these microbes that throw the digestive system further into disarray. These pathogens produce poisonous chemicals, creating more damage to the intestinal lining. For example, Candida albicans, a fungus, grows roots that invade and inflame the mucous lining of the intestines.[45]

The adrenals may become worn out from long-term production of cortisol, leading to adrenal fatigue, which manifests as exhaustion or chronic fatigue.[46]

Finally, cortisol decreases production of the *thyroid hormone carrier*, which prevents the body's cells from converting thyroid hormones T3 and T4. It also suppresses the secretion of a hormone called TSH in the pituitary gland. This prevents the thyroid from functioning properly.[47]

Cortisol Plays a Key Role in Disease Because It Regulates Inflammation

What are other important roles of cortisol? When the body becomes infected, proteins called cytokines are produced to trigger inflammation. Cytokines can be kept in check only by cortisol. The constant production of cortisol, however, causes bodily tissues to become less sensitive to its effects over time. This condition is known as *cortisol resistance* (similar to *insulin resistance* in the case of diabetes). Where there is cortisol resistance, the production of cytokines cannot be halted.[48]

Inflammation, as we mentioned in Chapter Two (page 49), is not a bad thing per se provided the body can utilize it to eliminate and detoxify. Chronic or uncontrolled inflammation, however, leads to symptoms like pain, lethargy and swelling. Basically, these are the symptoms that we call disease. In other words, chronic inflammation IS disease.

Stress, Cortisol and Unregulated Inflammation are Responsible for All Disease

Let's look at how cortisol and the associated hormones generated by stress can lead to different kinds of diseases.

Cortisol maintains blood glucose levels. [49] Another adrenal gland hormone called *epinephrine* turns off the release of insulin. [50] So cortisol resistance contributes to **High Blood Glucose** and the disease **Diabetes.**

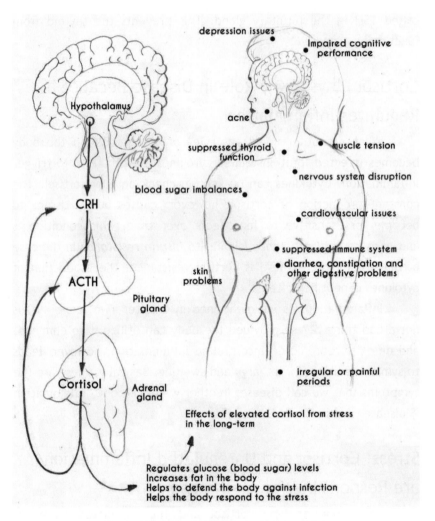

Figure 4: Effects of Stress on the Body

Cortisol affects the thyroid hormone that controls energy production in cells. High cortisol levels therefore cause less energy to be generated in the cells of the body. The liver works more sluggishly.

As a result, blood cholesterol is not converted by the liver into bile, leading to **High Cholesterol**.[51]

Another adrenal hormone adrenaline stimulates the cardiovascular and nervous systems, but chronically high levels of adrenaline elevate blood pressure and damage the heart muscle.[52] This is therefore a major contributor to **High Blood Pressure** and **Heart Diseases**. Persistently high levels of cortisol also cause a narrowing of the blood vessels, increasing the chance for a **Stroke**.[53]

As cortisol receptors are found in abundance in the hippocampus, a part of the brain, chronically elevated levels of cortisol causes the hippocampus to shrink. This is associated with **Cognitive Problems** like memory loss, concentration and focus issues.[54] This is also associated with diseases like **Parkinson's disease, Dementia** and **Alzheimer's disease**.

Cortisol depletes norepinephrine, the hormone responsible for energy and alertness, leading to **Chronic Fatigue**.[55]

Cortisol lowers the production of feel-good hormones such as dopamine and serotonin, which makes the organism vulnerable to all sorts of mood disorders, including **Depression, Anxiety** and **Suicidal Tendencies**.[56]

Cortisol affects the production of melatonin, an important hormone for regulating the sleep cycle. As a result, **Insomnia** develops.[57]

I can go on and on, but I've made the point: stress is the underlying cause for ALL disease and cortisol is its agent. In particular, stress adversely affects three main body systems.

In the hormonal system, the thyroid and adrenal glands become fatigued over time.

In the immune system, stress affects the spleen, thymus and lymph glands.

Finally in the digestive system, stress lacerates the intestinal lining.[58]

The combination of dysfunction in these three systems then leads to disease symptoms as we know them.

Summary

During stress, the HPA Axis gets activated. Hormones, especially cortisol, are released. If this stress response isn't turned off, the adrenals keep pumping out cortisol. Cortisol causes the three conditions seen in all chronic diseases: leaky gut syndrome, adrenal fatigue and thyroid issues. Over time, the body develops cortisol resistance. With cortisol resistance, the body can no longer control its production of cytokines; this then leads to widespread inflammation. Inflammation causes symptoms that manifest as different diseases, depending on where the inflammation is located in the body.

A number of studies have shown stress to be the underlying cause of ALL disease. For example, a cell biologist known as Bruce Lipton points out that physiological stress is the cause of at least 95 percent of diseases and conditions. (The remaining 5 percent is genetic; it is caused by stress somewhere in the ancestry of that person.[59])

According to convention, a disease is named or identified by its symptoms. That is how we differentiate between cancer, heart disease and Parkinson's disease, for example; they have different symptoms. But if all the different symptoms are simply a matter of stress manifesting in different forms, isn't it more accurate to say that there is only one true disease: stress?

Based on this argument, avoiding stress evidently is the way to prevent or heal all disease. Therefore, we must take a step back and ask why and when the stress response is activated.

FIVE — Traumas: The Basis of the Stress Response

The Stress Response is Natural in the Wild as a Means to Gain Mates and Territory

It's the mating season. Two male bears have locked eyes on each other. The duel between them will determine whether they get to stay on in the territory and mate with females in the area, or move on to fight another bear, another place, another day.

The bigger bear lifts itself up onto its hind legs and gives a roar befitting its dominant status. The other, seeing the aggression, cows down. The battle is over even before it began.

The loser slinks off into the trees; we soon lose sight of it. The winner, after checking to make sure its opponent is really gone, starts shaking vigorously. Calm after a while, it wanders off as well.

This scenario happens all the time in the wilds. Underneath the surface, however, a complex biochemistry of stress-related reactions occurs in the bodies of both these bears before, during and after the 'fight'.

Process of Stress involves the Stressor, the Brain that Gives Meaning to the Event, and the Stress Response

The process of stress has three parts to it. Firstly, an event happens that the animal finds threatening. This is known as the *stressor*. Secondly, there is a processing system that experiences and gives meaning to the event. This is in general the nervous system and in particular the brain. Finally, there is the *stress response*: the specific actions taken by the body as a reaction to the threat.[60]

In the example of the bears above, first each bear discovers the other bear in the territory. Secondly, each bear processes the experience and gives meaning to the event; if it interprets the experience as implying a threat to its ability to mate or survive, it has to ready itself for a fight. Finally, each bear's body responds with certain biochemical reactions, manifested (in the bigger bear) as the bear acting out its aggression and puffing itself up to look bigger and more threatening.

Our Nervous System, Especially Our Reptilian Brain, Decides Whether Something is a Threat

To understand how bears and humans process and give meaning to an event, we must look at a system known as our nervous system. Part of the nervous system is the central nervous system, consisting of our brain and spinal cord.

Paul MacLean, a neurobiologist, discovered that our brain is made up of three distinct parts, also called the *triune* brains:

1. The *reptilian* brain, technically known as the R-complex, which is instinctive and seeks to protect us from harm;[61]
2. The *mammalian* brain, technically known as the limbic brain, the part that causes us to feel emotions; and
3. The *neo-cortex*, our logical and reasoning part of the brain.

This structure corresponds to evolutionary theory: the first brain to develop was the reptilian brain, followed by the mammalian brain and finally the neo-cortex. (In case you're wondering: bears' brains are actually similar to ours except that their neo-cortex is not as developed.)

Due to the overwhelming drive for survival honed over millions of years of evolution (clearly not just of humans but of the evolutionary lineage that preceded us), our reptilian brain has become particularly reactive to possible threats from the environment. Any time the reptilian brain senses a potential threat it sends a signal along the *peripheral nervous system* (another part of the nervous system), consisting of neurons that convey impulses from our sensory organs — like our hands, fingers, toes, muscles and glands — to the central nervous system so that the body can process this information.

Here we are interested particularly in what we call the *autonomic nervous system*, the part of the peripheral nervous system which regulates involuntary bodily processes such as breathing, heart rate, digestion and metabolism. It consists of two sub-systems that are opposite in their effects.

Sympathetic System is activated during Stress and the Parasympathetic System during Relaxation

The *sympathetic nervous system* is activated in times of threat to present a 'fight or flight' response by accelerating bodily processes and protecting the body against potential damage. Conversely, the *parasympathetic nervous system* supports the 3Rs: rest, relax and rejuvenate.[62]

The sympathetic and parasympathetic systems (see figure below) are very much present in bears as well. If there is nothing threatening a bear, moving into the parasympathetic state is the natural state of its body. This state is known as the 'relaxation response'. However, when a threat is present — for example, when a bear senses a fight is imminent — its body moves into the sympathetic state. This state is known as the 'stress response'.

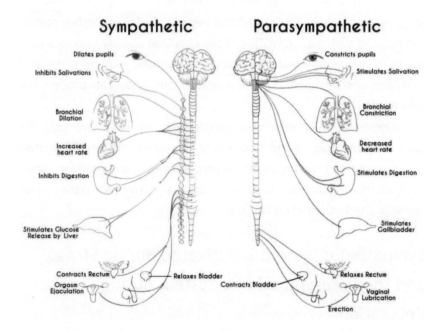

Figure 5: Sympathetic and Parasympathetic Systems

The Stress Response is Needed When There is a Threat to One's Life

Why is the stress response needed at all, for bear or man?

In a crisis in which a bear's survival is at stake, it is vital that the bear keeps its muscles strong. Hence blood flow has to be diverted to limbs like the arms and legs in preparation for fighting or escaping. Natural painkillers and blood-clotting resources need to be on standby in the event that there is an injury. It's like a country going into a state of emergency. All resources now need to be rationed and utilized for survival. Digestion, sexual functions, sleep and detoxification are all considered secondary functions and are prioritized lower than survival.[63]

In other words, stress response and detoxification are in fact inversely related. The more we are stressed, the less we detox, and vice versa. This, as we shall see later, has important implications for health.

Releasing Pent-Up Energy Brings the Body Out of a Stress Response

Let's return to our discussion of the bears. Whether a bear fights or runs away, the energy generated by going into the stress response gets expended. In our example, a mere display of aggression is enough to determine which bear is the dominant one. As a result, not all the energy generated is used up. That's why at the end the bear shakes it off; it's a way to release any 'left-over' energy. This allows the bear's body to come back to homeostasis as the body realizes that the threat is over. This is nature's way for animals to reset their stress response system.[64]

Humans are essentially animals; we have very similar nervous systems. Observe someone who is just coming out of shock and you may find her body naturally starting to shiver as a way to disperse the excess energy that was built up.

However, often times instead of helping someone process her experience we interrupt the process before it can come to completion because we do not understand that this is the body's way to return to its natural parasympathetic state.

The law of conservation of energy states that energy can neither be created nor destroyed; it can only change form. When the excess energy generated by stress has no outlet for dissipation, the energy becomes 'stuck' potential energy, and keeps us in the sympathetic stress response. I call this kind of event a trauma, because the body is not able to come back to its normal relaxation state.

Since Humans Think About Their Experiences, Even Perceived Threats, Not Just Actual Threats, Can Cause Traumas

Human stressors can differ from those of bears. Since we are born with the ability to reason, we tend to think about our situation and assign meanings to it, probably very unlike bears. Stress can arise from uncertainty, lack of information and a loss of control; these three factors represent the absence or threatened loss of something that we universally perceive as essential for survival.[65]

Our biology appears to make no distinction between an actual threat and the perception of a threat. Hence, stress can occur even when we are contemplating a future possibility (ie one that has not yet occurred). This can be uncertainty about the future, loss of income, financial problems, awaiting news concerning the life or death of loved ones, or being directly involved in a natural or man-made disaster.[66] In other words, traumas can occur not just because we are experiencing something that really threatens our life but also when we are simply *thinking* about a possible stressful experience.

Whether an Event is Traumatic or Not Depends on Our Initial Interpretation of the Event

Whether a threat is interpreted as traumatic or not seems to depend on the meaning we give to the event. Specifically, an event is traumatic if we make what is called a *Decision of Defeat*.[67]

Our goals, at different stages in life or different points in time, whether explicitly spoken of or implicitly intended, can be very different. For example, when a baby is born, the goal (implicit) can be as simple as being fed. The baby cries loudly to attract the attention of her mother, and becomes calm again when she gets to suckle on her mother's breast. In other words, our achievement of a goal obliterates the goal. That is, until the next goal surfaces in our consciousness. This happens constantly throughout our life.

In fact, our life can be summarized as a series of goals and actions to achieve those goals. At different points in our lives, we want different things: food, water, shelter, toys or cars. These needs are also not limited to the physical. We also have emotional needs such as love and touch. In our drive to meet our needs, we may experience obstacles; needs may sometimes not get met. The child who did not get the ice cream despite throwing a tantrum; the man who did not get the woman he wanted as his lover; the woman who failed to get her job promotion: all these are examples of our goals being thwarted.

When these events happen, the crucial factor is the meaning we assign these experiences. We can make a Decision of Defeat: "My parents don't love me enough to get me an ice-cream", "I am unlovable", or "I am a failure". Or we can make a *Decision of Grace*: we can choose to see the experience in a positive way, as an experience to learn from in achieving other goals in future.

The choice we make — a Decision of Defeat or a Decision of Grace — is crucial. The same 'negative' experience can be interpreted in two different ways by two persons making different choices. This choice subsequently affects how each person's body responds to the incident, whether with a stress or relaxation response. In other words, *an event becomes a trauma only when there is a Decision of Defeat attached to it*, and our interpretation of this event as a trauma is then what causes us to react with stress to it.

Repressing Emotions Can be Deadly

When we choose, because of unmet goals, to make a Decision of Defeat, we also feel the emotions associated with that thought.

A child who does not get the ice-cream he wanted may make a Decision of Defeat — that he wasn't loved by his parents — and would probably feel a mix of emotions, like anger and sadness. He may throw a tantrum in a bid to get his way. The father may hush him up with a warning: "You had better stop now or I am going to give you a thrashing." The boy now has to bottle up all the anger and sadness that he is feeling to avoid a beating. These emotions become repressed.

5 - Traumas: The Basis of the Stress Response

To illustrate how harmful chronic emotional repression is, let's look at Cvrenka, a small town in the former republic of Yugoslavia, in the years 1965-1966.

During this period, one thousand men and four hundred women, all of whom did not manifest any symptoms of disease at the beginning, were selected from this town to fill in a 109-item questionnaire that measured both emotional and personality characteristics as well as physical measures like weight, blood pressure and smoking history. Ten years later, in 1976, over 40 percent of these 1,400 people had died, from heart conditions, cancer and other causes. The biggest risk factor for death from cancer turned out to be the repression of anger.

On closer inspection of one of the cancers — lung cancer — something even more surprising emerged.

One would have expected participants who were smokers to be at much higher risk of developing lung cancer. This was true: every single person who had lung cancer was a smoker. However, it also turned out that tobacco smoke was a risk factor for cancer only for those people who were also emotionally repressed. All those who succumbed to lung cancer had high scores when it came to repressing their anger. Those who didn't could apparently smoke packs of cigarettes without getting lung cancer![68]

Remember how bears reset their stress response by shaking? Repressing emotion is the equivalent of not allowing the excess energy that was built up to be released. It gets stuck inside the body and keeps us in the stressed state. That's why we feel so much better after a good cry. The pent-up emotions built up in our body are released, allowing the body to move more completely into a relaxation state.

I mentioned earlier how stress is inversely related to detoxification. Could you now understand why repression of emotions is a major contributing factor in illnesses like cancer? Apparently, whether a person is able to remove toxins is a function not just of how much toxins she is exposed to (in the Cvrenka study, how much cigarettes she smoked) but also of whether she has the habit of repressing her emotions.

Illness seems to have two components. Firstly, there has to be a physical component: the toxins we mentioned. Secondly, there must be an emotional component, which seems to be more important than the physical component. The emotional component determines whether the toxins stay in the body to poison us, or whether the body finds a way to purge them from the system.

Summary

All animals, including humans, are always trying to maintain a state of homeostasis. When we are exposed to any stressors — be they physical (physical threat to safety), chemical (exposure to foreign substances), biological (physical injuries, on-going infections) or even psychological (phobias) — our stress response get activated if we interpret the event as a threat. The heart pumps faster; more blood is channeled to the muscles to mount an effective 'fight or flight' response.

The stress response is actually an attempt by our body to maintain homeostasis in the face of the threat, so that we may continue to function safely. In an era of natural predators and other dangers, this stress response was indispensable for survival. In our current age, it is often triggered in situations where it is neither necessary nor helpful. We create our own meanings for our experiences. Specifically, we may make Decisions of Defeat in response to the traumas we experience, and then suppress these emotions so that our body never goes completely back to the relaxation state.

While acute stress is the immediate, short-term bodily response to threat, chronic stress entails activation of the stress mechanisms over long periods of time. It's chronic stress that we look to for explanation of our chronic illness, ie when our body is no longer able to detox properly.

Now that we understand what traumas are and how they can affect our health, let's examine another related question: does it matter when these traumas happen?

SIX — Current Life: How Our Health in Adulthood is shaped by Birth and Childhood Traumas

Emotional Repression Traits Could Start From Childhood

Tiffany is my client. She is in her early 60s, mild-mannered, and displays few emotions. She also suffers from stomach cancer. Towards the end of one of her therapy sessions with me, we were casually chatting when she told me her story.

Tiffany's father was very strict with her, from a very young age. She was even physically abused by him during childhood. This continued until her teens. She recalled one incident when, as a teenager, she got into an argument with her father. In a fit of anger, he pushed her down on the chair, took out his belt and started whipping her. Her mother, powerless to do anything, could only look on.

After the thrashing, Tiffany couldn't even stand up let alone walk properly. She took to bed for almost a month. Recovery was slow but she eventually regained her ability to walk.

This wasn't the first time she had been beaten so severely (and it wouldn't be the last). This incident got burned into her memory because it was the most severe beating of the many she received. The irony is that today she can't even recall what they were arguing about.

In the previous chapter, I mentioned how repressed emotions can lead to disease later on. Tiffany's emotional repression started in her childhood and became a habit in her adulthood. To understand how emotional repression can become ingrained, let's go back to the triune brain.

Current Events are Interpreted According to Association with Past Threats

In the triune brain, the neo-cortex is the only part of the brain that works with rational thought. Both the mammalian and reptilian brains work mainly with associations. For example, the scent of a particular perfume may remind you of a lover you once had, or eating a certain food can bring back fond memories of mum's cooking.

Similarly, all the feelings, thoughts, sensations, sounds and images that Tiffany experienced as a result of the traumatic beatings she received in her childhood were encoded in her mind as strong memories.

In Tiffany's adulthood, similar feelings, thoughts, sensations, sounds or images that even remotely remind her reptilian brain of these past traumas will activate, through association, a stress response in Tiffany.

Unfortunately, the way our mind associates memories can often work against us.

We Have Coping Mechanisms Because of Past Hurts, but These May No Longer Be Rational When Considering Current Circumstances

The reptilian brain is the first part of the triune brain to develop. As such, especially in the first six years of life when the neo-cortex is not yet fully developed, all memories of an incident are interpreted by the individual's reptilian brain based on the thinking ability of the individual at the time the incident occurred.

As an adult we can use our neo-cortex brain to rationalize, but as a child we do not have that ability. In other words, as a child we could well have made a Decision of Defeat (Chapter 5, page 87), since we did not, at that age, have the ability to interpret the experience logically. As a result, we react to present traumas with coping behavior that may have been appropriate for the threat at a point in the past but which is irrational when viewed in the current situation.

For example, people who know Tiffany consider her a 'nice lady', but her niceness is actually a coping mechanism, from childhood, meant to avoid her father's rage.

Every time she hears someone raise his voice, her mind immediately associates that with the physical abuse she endured as a child. Tiffany becomes once again the little girl who couldn't protect herself, even though she's now a grown woman.

As a result, an internal conflict tears at her. At one level, she feels anger whenever her boundaries are breached by others; at another level, she feels compelled to repress this anger because, based on the logic of her reptilian brain, to express it would lead only to physical assault. Tiffany thus never asserts herself and allows others to take advantage of her.

Our Personality is shaped by Our Unconscious Coping Mechanisms

Logically, Tiffany may know the right thing to do, but she's unable to do it because of the associations in her reptilian brain. She is literally hard wiring that *stimulus response* into her nervous system every time she reacts unconsciously. This forms her thinking and emotional habits which, with time and practice, becomes her personality. The more it gets hard-wired into her system, the harder it is for her to change it.[69]

That, by the way, is also how all of us behave as adults. The mammalian and reptilian brains, our unconscious minds, have been shown to be millions of times more powerful than the neo-cortex, our conscious mind.[70] This is not surprising considering that the reptilian brain is involved in all the unconscious functions of our body. Imagine what life would be like if you had to consciously make your heart beat or your hair grow.

As a result, it is not our conscious beliefs that hold sway as adults. We often make decisions based on our instinctive urges (from the reptilian brain) and emotions (from the mammalian brain). With time, we even rationalize our decisions, saying we made a logical decision based on the facts at hand, when the opposite was actually true: we made a decision unconsciously and then justified it logically.

We Often Unconsciously Repress Our Trauma Memories

Let's return to Tiffany's story, to illustrate how easy it can be to rationalize our decisions when in reality they stem from repressed trauma memories.

On one of Tiffany's therapy sessions, we got to talking about forgiveness. I mentioned that lack of forgiveness towards someone in life appeared to be a consistent theme in the life of the cancer clients I had seen.

Tiffany responded that there was no one in her life that she hadn't forgiven. I let the matter slide; it wasn't the time to pursue it further.

Tiffany then mentioned how her mother, Yvonne, had never really loved her father, Tim. Yvonne passed away before Tim. At her deathbed, Yvonne made Tiffany promise that she would not be buried together with Tim in their ancestral home in China.

After the death of her mother, Tiffany had a huge argument with her father on the matter. Tiffany told him of Yvonne's clear instructions not to be buried together with him, but Tim was adamant about bringing Yvonne's remains back to China. Tiffany admitted defeat; when her father finally passed away, he was buried next to his wife in China.

The entire episode was so ugly that Tiffany refused to go back to China to pay her respect at the tombs of her parents, despite repeated calls by her siblings to do so.

"I will never go back to China to see my father because he didn't respect the wishes of my mother. Furthermore, I can't bear to face my mother because I couldn't keep the promise I made to her."

She said that in a calm tone, but you can probably imagine the immense amount of pain that she was suppressing inside. It was clear from her story that Tiffany did indeed have people in her life she couldn't forgive: her father ... and herself.

Although she wasn't able to forgive either herself or her father, she wasn't aware of this: she had suppressed those feelings so much that to her conscious mind, there was no problem at all.

Tiffany's dramatic story illustrates a common truth. Many people are not aware that they have suffered traumatic experiences because they have repressed their feelings so as to continue functioning in life. At some point, those repressed feelings manifest as disease.

In fact, a study has shown that 90 percent of people who indicated that they don't feel stressed were found to be so when a test was done to determine how much cortisol was present in their blood, indicating how stressed they truly were.[71]

The More Severe Our Traumas, The More We Are Affected by It, and The More We Repress Our Memories of it

The more severe the trauma the stronger its impact on our psyche; at the same time, ironically, the more we subconsciously try to avoid similar experiences in future and the more we repress our memories of it.

Tiffany's severe traumas related to her father meant that she tended to be more cautious with authority figures; that would be the advance warning her reptilian brain would give her, based on her past negative experiences. She also felt a strong sense of unease, without knowing why, in the presence of these people. (She didn't know because the association to these past threats had already become unconscious.)

Try this experiment: go into a room where the air-conditioner is on. Initially when you go into the room, you can hear the sound of the air-conditioner humming. After a while, as you busy yourself with work, the humming fades into the background and you no longer have conscious awareness of it.

If we had to assimilate all the stimuli from the environment all the time, we would certainly become overwhelmed. Hence, the body allows us to be consciously aware of only a tiny fraction of everything happening around us.

We tend to notice only the things that are changing. In our air-conditioner example, your conscious awareness of the sound coming from the unit would probably be triggered again if someone came into the room and switched it off. All of a sudden, the humming stops; you register that as a change of sound. If things don't change, we become insensitive to them after a while. In fact, this process of desensitization is happening to us all the time so that we can adapt to everything around us.

If we kept re-experiencing all the traumas that we had ever experienced, life would quickly become too painful for us. At the same time, we cannot forget them: these traumas left painful memories. Hence, the reptilian brain — which is biologically geared to survival — is on constant guard, sending you signals through the stress response to avoid experiencing these traumas again.

6 – Current Life: How Our Health in Adulthood is Shaped by Birth and Childhood Traumas

The only way to reconcile these opposing considerations is for these traumatic experiences to become unconscious. You no longer consciously remember all the painful traumatic memories from the past; after a while you become desensitized to them the same way you stop noticing the humming sound from the air-conditioner — until it stops. Your reptilian brain, however, doesn't stop scanning the environment, even if you are not consciously aware of this.

This explains all the irrational fears of people, ie why people are afraid of enclosed spaces, height, spiders, snakes, water, etc. The mind has associated these things to memories about experiences in the past when these things represented danger to life.

This phenomenon is especially pronounced in *Post-Traumatic Stress Disorder* (PTSD), a condition in which people who experienced a shock as a result of an overwhelming event continue to suffer unpleasant recollections of the incident. Veterans of the Vietnam War, fought between the US and South Vietnam on one side and North Vietnam and China on the other, in the period 1955-1975, often felt a jarring shock when they heard a loud sound even many years after the war. In their mind, loud sounds were a reminder of the risk they constantly faced on the battlefield from guns, bombs and enemy combatants. Years after the war their body would still associate a sudden loud sound with a life and death situation.

As these examples show, the reptilian brain does not understand the concept of time. A trauma may have occurred many years ago; the reptilian brain, however, believes it is still happening.

The Earlier the Trauma, the Stronger its Present Effect

We have mentioned that the reptilian brain works on associations, meaning that later memories must be associated with earlier ones. This logically implies that earlier traumas should affect us more. In fact, based on clinical observations, they do.[72] (Just as logically, the more severe the trauma is, the stronger the later effect will be.)

Stanislav Grof, a Czech psychiatrist, coined the term *Systems of Condensed Experiences* (COEX) to describe this chain of associated memories. In brief, memories of the same kind are grouped together by association, with the earliest trauma being the most pivotal. Later memories involving a similar emotion are added onto the COEX structure as and when experienced.[73]

Because of this, I am not an advocate of positive thinking alone, ie that we can consciously 'think ourselves' to health. Our challenges, stresses, responses, etc, are not just the result of our conscious thoughts but the deep unconscious structures in the COEX.

So when, do you think, are the earliest memories you have from this current life that can possibly affect you?

If you answered 'birth', you would be right. Let's go back to the time when we were just a fetus in our mother's womb.

Since the Earliest and Most Severe Traumas are Birth Traumas, They Have a Profound Impact on Our Personality and Health

Prenatal and perinatal psychologists generally agree that a fetus in the womb already has awareness of its environment and can feel pain (there are disagreements on when exactly this occurs).

Consciousness definitely arises way before birth. In fact, during pregnancy, the baby believes that all emotions experienced by the mother are being experienced by it *itself*. Hence, any emotional stress experienced by the mother can adversely affect the developing fetus. Some studies have shown that some adult complexes can actually be traced back to emotions experienced by the mother while the fetus was in her womb.[74]

This is NOT the conventional, mainstream view. Traditional medical practitioners believe that the cerebral cortex of the newborn is not fully *myelinated* — meaning that the neurons in the brain are not yet fully covered with a protective layer of fat called *myelin* — at birth. This means, according to them, that infants are incapable of recording their womb or birth memories.

This sounds illogical to me: even 'lower' life forms that do not have a cerebral cortex have demonstrated that they have memory mechanisms. For example, Swedish physiologist Eric Kandel got the 2000 Nobel Prize in Medicine for studying how a sea slug's memory system works.[75]

The memory mechanism that allows even babies to record memories will be explored further in Chapter Seven.

6 – Current Life: How Our Health in Adulthood is Shaped by Birth and Childhood Traumas

If womb and birth memories *can be* recorded by the developing fetus, what are the implications?

During birth, the human baby — with a head disproportionately large, due to the size of the human brain, compared to the rest of its body — comes out of its mother's body through a narrow birth canal. This means that birth is a difficult and painful process for both mother and child.

(The human birth canal has to be narrow otherwise women would have a pelvis that is too wide for them to stand upright. Furthermore, the human species is the only one on the planet in which the baby rotates, inside the womb, from a head-up position to a head-down position at full term, in order to be born.)

A fetus in the womb is biologically programmed to know when to activate its birth process, travel through the canal, and induce a number of biochemical hormones, in an act of supreme cooperation with the mother so as to make delivery possible.

Any interruption of this process can be harmful, stressful and traumatic to the baby. For example, cases of induced birth, caesarean delivery, or delivery due to forceps or suction can be traumatic to the baby.[76]

During birth, a fetus experiences some of the most excruciating pain that it will typically ever experience in its life. In fact, almost no babies come out unscathed, the difference in the trauma experienced being only a matter of degree.

Now recall that we stated that the earlier the trauma an individual experiences, the stronger its effect on the individual in later life. Since biological birth is one of the earliest and most profound traumas in life, it forms the basis for many of our strongest personality traits and health issues.[77]

So is there any scientific research that shows that early incidents, whether in birth or childhood, can cause disease? Indeed there is.

Research is Showing that Adverse Childhood Incidents Can Cause Diseases Later On in Life

In the 1980s, Dr. Vincent Felitti was trying to help severely obese people lose weight by getting them to do a liquid diet. It worked like a charm: grossly obese patients who were able to do it for a year could lose as much as 135 kg!

Then he discovered that the people who couldn't maintain the liquid diet and reverted to their normal diets gained all their weight back very quickly, sometimes even faster than they had lost it.

Perplexed, he started studying the backgrounds of the participants of his program, and found that more than half of his three hundred participants had been sexually abused as children! This was clearly way above the average of the general population. Dr. Felitti became convinced that there was a direct cause between childhood sexual abuse and severe obesity in adulthood.[78] He decided to explore further. Could there be links between childhood traumas and other disease conditions in adulthood?

The result was the Adverse Childhood Experiences (ACE) study, with over 17,000 participants, one of the largest such studies ever conducted. The results were shocking.

The study found that ACE was strongly associated with addictions, alcoholism, depression, heart disease, liver disease, suicide and post-traumatic stress disorders, amongst many others. Since then, many other studies have corroborated these results.[79]

The link between sexual abuse in childhood and obesity in adulthood that Dr. Felitti found offers an intriguing possibility: could the abused person be unconsciously shaping her body to become as unattractive as possible to avoid the risk and/or trauma of sexual abuse? This hypothesis is well in line with our other hypothesis that our consciousness shapes our physical body (Chapter Three, page 62).

This begs a related question: if diseases are caused by stress, and stress is activated by traumas, why are there different manifestations of stress for different individuals? Is there a relationship between the traumas that a person experiences and the diseases they subsequently contract?

In other words, what determines what disease(s) a person who is subject to chronic stress develops?

The Symptoms we Manifest Depend on Our Specific Emotional Vulnerabilities

We often use metaphors to describe how we feel. For example, we talk about 'butterflies in the stomach', 'a pain in the neck' or 'feeling pissed off'.

It's interesting, and no coincidence, that the terms we use tying emotions to body organs are borne out by many ancient traditions, for example TCM.

'Butterflies in the stomach' represents anxiety; ancient traditions or holistic practitioners have long depicted anxiety as an emotion generated by the stomach. Similarly, whenever someone comes to me complaining of a persistent 'pain in the neck' –

metaphorically meaning an annoying person — I invariably find that there is someone present at that point in her life that she finds annoying. Similarly, 'feeling pissed off' (irritation) often manifests as a problem in the bladder.

The table below lists a few of these Organ-Emotion links.

Organ/Area Dysfunctions	Emotions
Adrenals	Fright and exhaustion
Arms	Reaching out for support and not getting it
Back, Lower	Financial worries and concerns
Back, Upper	Holding back love
Bladder	Irritation
Brain	Loss of control
Ears	Not being listened to
Eyes	Not wanting to see something
Gallbladder	Resentment
Heart	Lack of love and connection
Hips	Lack of support
Intestines, Small	Neglect, abandonment or loneliness
Intestines, Large	Being over-critical

Organ/Area Dysfunctions	Emotions
Kidneys	Fear
Legs	Not knowing how to move forward
Liver	Anger
Lungs	Grief and sadness
Neck	Annoyance by someone or something
Pancreas	Lack of joy
Sexual organs	Guilt and shame
Shoulders	Heavy responsibility
Spleen	Low self-esteem/indecisiveness
Stomach	Anxiety
Thymus	Self-protection
Thyroid	Communication/expression issues

There is a 'right-left divide' as well.

The right side of our body is controlled by the left hemisphere of our brain, which is associated with our masculine and logical side. The left side of our body is controlled by the right hemisphere of our brain, which is associated with our feminine and intuitive side.

6 – Current Life: How Our Health in Adulthood is Shaped by Birth and Childhood Traumas

Physical issues on the right side of the body are associated with concerns over career and money while issues on the left side of the body are associated with concerns over relationships.

Here are practical examples of how I use these relationships.

If someone comes to me with pain in the left knee I check with them if they have concerns about moving forward in a relationship. With someone who complains of pain in the right ear, I usually ask if he feels that he is not being listened to at work.

In complex diseases like multiple sclerosis (MS), the metaphor principle is also a useful one to bear in mind. The main problem with MS patients is the loss of control of their body. This is usually related to a feeling of loss of control of their life, or a need to get it under control. Studies have shown that MS patients had experienced threatening events ten times more often and marital conflict five times more frequently than healthy control participants.[80]

Remember Tiffany (page 93)? Since she has cancer of the stomach, I would surmise that her dominant emotional vulnerability was actually anxiety.

An Austrian oncologist, Dr. Geerd Ryke Hamer, used a technology known as *computer tomography* to scan the brains of over 10,000 cancer patients. He found brain damage manifesting as light and dark dots in different parts of the brain; the locations corresponded to the type of traumas experienced.

These cancer patients had experienced trauma, mostly emotional in nature, which had left an indelible mark on their brain; in time, the trauma triggered cancer. When these emotional traumas were resolved, these marks in the brain disappeared.[81] (Dr. Hamer maintains a practice in Rome, Italy, treating cancer patients.)

6 – Current Life: How Our Health in Adulthood is Shaped by Birth and Childhood Traumas

I theorize that if Tiffany were to see Dr. Hamer, her computer tomography scan results would show marks in the part of the brain corresponding to the stomach, which is where her cancer – the result of the traumas she experienced with her father – would eventually manifest.

Emotions and their link to disease have been demonstrated in other large-scale studies.

Dr. Hans Jurgen Eysenck, a German psychologist, conducted a twenty-year study of over 13,000 European subjects and classified them according to four personality types:

1. The first group has a pattern of feeling hopelessness;
2. The second group feels blame or anger;
3. The third group alternates between both hopelessness and anger;
4. The fourth group takes responsibility for their own happiness.

Eysenck found that:

*   9 percent of people in the third group die of cancer or heart disease, while less than 1 percent of people in the fourth group die of these two diseases.
*   75 percent of people who die of heart disease and 15 percent of those who die of cancer come from the second group of people (those who are perpetually angry).
*   In group one (those who feel hopelessness), 75 percent eventually die of cancer and 15 percent from heart disease.[82]

We can use the metaphor of the weakest link to describe how this association between emotions, and the organs or areas of the body affected, comes about. Stress may affect the body equally, but it's the weakest link that breaks.

Someone who sprains his lower back when bending down to pick up his haversack from the floor may have been holding worries over financial matters in his consciousness for a long period of time.

In turn, these worries may have been thought patterns generated from Decisions of Defeat made as a result of past traumas. These thoughts and emotions, perhaps held for a long period of time or very powerful in their intensity, weaken the corresponding area of the body so that an external environmental trigger subsequently sparks off the physical problem.

This explains how our environment can shape our health. We cover how other environmental triggers set off diseases in more detail in Chapter Fourteen.

Summary

In the previous chapter, we found that Decisions of Defeat and the corresponding emotional repression are responsible for keeping us in a stressed response state that is subsequently responsible for disease.

In this chapter, we found that many of these thought and emotional patterns could be traced to birth and childhood – especially the period before six years of age, when experiences are interpreted by the reptilian brain, which works based on association instead of logic.

6 – Current Life: How Our Health in Adulthood is Shaped by Birth and Childhood Traumas

The earlier or more severe the trauma, the greater the impact it tends to have on our adult life. This means that by adulthood, we may have a personality that is already largely shaped by unconscious coping behavior patterns based on threats we experienced in the womb or in childhood.

Because of how painful these traumas can be, we also unconsciously repress the memories of these traumas. This means:

a. We are stressed and have no idea why; or

b. We are stressed and believe it is some external trigger (eg, your boss or your boyfriend) that is causing it, when this trigger merely set off a chain of associations from much earlier in our life; or

c. We think we are not stressed but we actually are. We have unconsciously repressed the trauma and think everything is fine, until we eventually succumb to an illness out of the blue.

You may be wondering how it is possible that the body can continue to activate the stress response for an event that has occurred in the past — in many cases, during childhood or even before. What about the adage "Time heals all wounds"?

I submit that this saying is not true. Somehow the body must retain a memory of the initial incident, and somehow this memory must still be affecting the body in the present, otherwise an illness would resolve itself with time.

Indeed, your body appears to hold all the memories you have ever experienced. This idea is explored in the next chapter.

SEVEN — Memories: Our Future is a Repeat of Our Past

Heart Transplant Brings Up the Question of Cellular Memories

In 1988, a US dancer called Claire Sylvia received a heart transplant from an 18-year-old male who had just died in a motorcycle accident. After she recovered from the surgery, she suddenly developed a voracious appetite for chicken nuggets, green peppers and beer. She had not been drawn to these foods before.

In addition, she started having a recurring dream about a man, Tim L., whom she'd never met. Believing that the man was linked to the donor of the heart now keeping her alive, she began a search to find out his identity. Eventually she located the family of the donor and discovered that his name was indeed Tim, and that he loved chicken nuggets, green peppers and beer.[83]

Claire's experience, as well as those of other patients who have experienced profound personality changes after an organ transplant, has opened up an inquiry into the idea of *cellular memory*. Can memories and personality traits be carried in the cells of the body and passed on to another person, even though the individual to whom these memories belonged was no longer alive?

Mainstream science does not allow for the possibility of cellular memory; memories are thought to be contained, in their entirety, in our brains, specifically in the area called the hippocampus. However, the truth is that despite a century of research, no one has managed to pin down the physical base of memories in the brain. Perhaps there is a very simple reason for this: memories are not found in the brain after all.

Memories Are Not Found in Our Brain

A US psychologist called Karl Lashley conducted a series of experiments on rats, monkeys and chimpanzees. He started by training the animals to perform various tasks ranging from the simple to the complex. After the training, he surgically removed parts of their brain, while keeping the animals alive, and observed what happened to the animals' memories. Even after large amounts of the brain had been removed, the animals could still remember how to perform those tasks. He concluded that memory cannot be localized to any part of the brain.[84]

The same phenomenon has been observed in a group of people who suffered from *hydrocephalus*, also known as 'water on the brain'. This condition is characterized by fluid in the skull. Some people found to have extreme hydrocephalus were surprisingly normal.

One young man in particular had an IQ of 126, and gained a first-class degree in Mathematics, yet he had just a thin layer, about a millimeter thick, of brain cells; the rest of his skull was filled with fluid. With a brain having only about 5 percent of the volume of the typical human brain, he was able to function remarkably well.

This begs the question as to whether the brain is really necessary at all.[85]

Could the Brain be Holographic?

Another psychologist, Karl Pribam from the United States, came to the conclusion that the brain had to be *holographic*; this was the only way to explain the mystery of how large amounts of neural tissue could be removed without affecting memory.

'Holographic' derives from the word 'hologram'. A hologram is a three-dimensional (3D) image created by the interference of light beams from a coherent light source, typically a laser. The image is recorded on a film. With just one beam of light to provide illumination, the film looks odd, showing patterns that look like water stains. However, with a second beam to illuminate the film, 3D images of the filmed object appear.

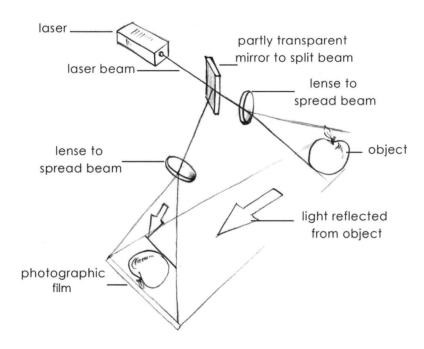

Figure 6: Creating a Hologram

Holographic images, unlike normal images, have a very special characteristic. Clearly, recording an object on film stores visual information about that image; this much we expect. What we wouldn't expect, however, is that a small piece of this film, cut out from the original, would still contain the image of the whole object (when shined on by the two laser beams)! To put it more generally, small sections of a film of a holographic image contain the same information as the entire film. (In very small sections of the film, though, the image does start to lose some of its clarity.)

Brains of humans (and other animals) have the same quality: even if I cut away large portions of the brain, the memories still remain.[86]

Now it's not just our brain that's been found to be holographic: physicists are finding that the entire universe seems to function as a hologram.[87]

Cellular Memories Exist

What is the implication of that last sentence? *A small part of the whole contains the whole.*

If a small part of the whole contains the whole, then is it possible that each cell of our body 'contains' information on the entire universe?

If the body is indeed a hologram, then each cell of the body contains information of the whole body. If there is a mechanism by which the body as a whole retains memories, each cell of the body also contains this memory. Since we know we have memories, if the body is a hologram this would therefore mean that cellular memories *must* exist.

Some scientists do believe in the notion of cellular memory. I'll highlight one here: American neuroscientist Dr. Candace Pert.

Dr. Pert achieved significant fame in the scientific community when she discovered the brain's *opiate* receptor; this is where *endorphins*, the feel-good hormones, bind to. Her research showed a *causal link* between our mind and body — ie, that one affects the other — and that cellular memory plays a big part in this link.

In the body, she found small proteins known as *neuropeptides* that can bind to receptors in cells. Whether you feel angry, sad or happy depends on your neuropeptides. These neuropeptides are thus the biochemical equivalent of emotions, and how they work is by accessing cellular memories stored throughout the body.

Neuropeptides have been found to play a significant role in switching *genes* on and off (genes are the part of our DNA that code for proteins; we explore this further when we discuss genetics in Chapter Eight and epigenetics in Chapter Nine).[88]

Again, the existence of neuropeptides shows a connection between our emotions and diseases, by showing how our emotions can affect the expression of our genes, and therefore lead to diseases.

Are cellular memories actually stored in 'physical storage areas' in cells? Mainstream scientists are reluctant to accept the cellular memory hypothesis because the mechanism showing how cells can store memories is currently not known.

Well, I believe the answer is to be found in the deepest recesses of our cells: our DNA.

Cellular Memories Could Be Stored in the DNA

In the field of Information Technology (IT), one of the greatest challenges has always been to find a medium that can store as much data as possible in the smallest space possible, for the longest time possible.

We have now found the solution. It's DNA.

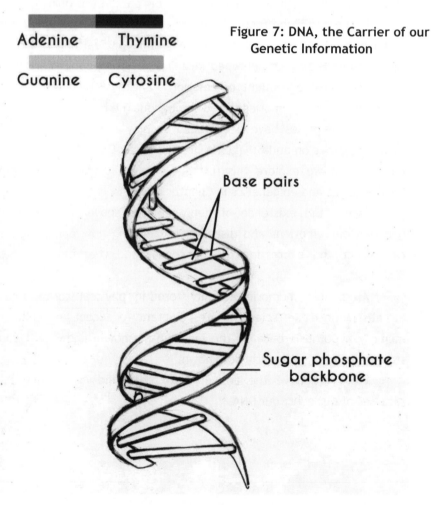

Adenine   Thymine

Guanine   Cytosine

Figure 7: DNA, the Carrier of our Genetic Information

Base pairs

Sugar phosphate backbone

DNA, *DeoxyriboNucleic Acid*, is self-replicating material found in nearly all living organisms. It is the carrier of genetic information, and the main constituent of chromosomes.

Apparently, the coding language of nature is very similar to how we code information in computers, except that DNA codes in terms of four nucleotides (basic structural units or 'letters') while conventional computers use a *binary code system* of 1 and 0.

In 2015, a study found that 28 grams of DNA molecules, which weighs less than a penny (the US 1-cent coin), could store 300,000 terabytes of information for at least a million years![89] (One terabyte, simplified, is a million million bytes, or 1,000,000,000,000 bytes.)

Do you believe this is a mere coincidence? I certainly don't think so. Nature has created DNA for a purpose. We know for sure that DNA codes for proteins in the physical body. By implication, DNA must contain information (organized data) on how to create a protein.

Think about a recent memory you had. Play back the images in your mind, the sensations in your body, the feelings and thoughts you were having that moment. Images, sensations, feelings, thoughts: all this is just information.

Why we love movies so much is because movies are the closest things to our memories, except they are on a flat screen instead of 3-dimensional (3D).

Nowadays, we can download movies because they can be digitized into data and stored in computers. Since we can store movies as digital information in computers, is it possible that our DNA similarly stores memories? Could DNA actually be a storage device for all the memories we have ever collected, just like our computer hard-disk stores movie and video data?

I'll go further: I believe DNA stores not just our individual memories but the memories of *everything that has ever happened in the evolution of all living things*. This includes memories of our own ancestors; memories of people we've never met, from eras long before ours; and even the memories of the ancient, distant dinosaurs we may well be descended from.

But as always, the physical mechanisms of memory explain only part of the story. I would now like to explore the non-physical aspects of memory.

Morphic Resonance Explains How Living Things Can Tap into a Collective Field

Every year, monarch butterflies make a mass migration from Canada to Central Mexico to hibernate for the winter and then return for the summer.

Here's the interesting thing: the journey, of about 5,900 miles (9,495 kilometers), from Canada to Mexico and back is far too long for any single butterfly to complete. It takes *three to five generations of butterflies over the course of a year* to make the entire trip.[90]

Therein lies a huge mystery: how is it possible that the butterflies retain the 'memory' of where they should migrate to and what route they should take when no single butterfly lives long enough to have that memory in its DNA? This mystery has puzzled scientists for a long time.

Rupert Sheldrake, a British biologist, believes he has the answer: *morphic resonance*.

The concept came about from some interesting findings that Sheldrake discovered in laboratories across the world, ranging from Harvard in the United Kingdom to universities in Melbourne, Australia.

Sheldrake found that when rats were first exposed to a new maze, they took a long time to figure out how to escape from it. This isn't at all surprising; clearly, there must be a learning curve for something new.

What was mind-boggling was that if rats in one location learned how to maneuver through a maze, rats in other places seemed to learn the solution much faster, even though these different groups of rats had no contact whatsoever.

Could the learning have come about through genetics? The answer was no. Firstly, many of these rats were not even linked ancestrally. Secondly, even rats with parents that had never been trained to escape the maze were found to improve as quickly as those with parents that were trained.[91]

Another anomalous result was found in Intelligence Quotient (IQ) testing. Average IQ test scores have risen by 30 per cent or more since IQ tests came into vogue. This has been attributed to people becoming more intelligent because of better diet, but could it also be that as more people answer IQ questions, the 'memory' of their answers makes it easier for people coming after to answer these questions?[92]

All this sounds like the stuff of science fiction unless we consider the premise of morphic resonance. Resonance is how one object that is vibrating can cause or influence another to vibrate. For example, if a swinging pendulum is introduced into a room of stationary pendulums, eventually all the pendulums will become synchronized and swing at the same rate.

In quantum physics we have a model known as Super Strings Theory (SST) that asserts that strings are the most basic subatomic unit of matter, ie that everything around us is made of strings.

Strings are thought to be vibrating all the time, so all of us are made up of continually vibrating strings. Just like the first pendulum in our example above causes all the other pendulums to synchronize with it, we are all also in partial resonance with each other.

Everything is resonating with everything else across space and time. The more similar two things are, the more they resonate with each other.[93]

This is the basis for the well-known Law of Attraction (LOA), a term that came into vogue with the movie *The Secret*. In brief, LOA states that the thoughts you hold in your head will eventually create your reality, based on the principle that like (thoughts) attracts like (reality).

Memories are Stored in this Collective Field, Also Known as the Morphogenetic Field

If the vibration of a string that was originally in sync with other strings is changed, two things can happen.

The first possibility is that the other strings can change to match the string that was changed. This usually happens when a 'critical mass' is reached.

The second possibility is that the other strings can 'help' the string that was changed to return to its initial vibration.

The first possibility is very similar to the idea of a *tipping point*, the idea that if sufficient people believe in a certain idea, product or service, all of a sudden a paradigm shift happens and the product or service becomes accepted as part of the mainstream.

The second effect explains inertia — the reason habits can be so very hard to break. Over the long term, change inevitably happens; however, on a day-to-day basis, when we look at ourselves, very little seems to change: our appearance appears to be more-or-less the same.

Based on the idea of morphic resonance, we maintain our individual identity by resonating with our past. By resonating with our past, we also tap into a field of collective memories generated from all those who have come before who have experienced similar events as us. Our rate of learning is faster than that of our predecessors because we are not just learning afresh but drawing upon their experiences and adding to it.[94]

This would explain why monarch butterflies can find their hibernating grounds: the butterflies are in morphic resonance with their ancestors who made a similar trip.

Morphic resonance would explain why once some rats have learnt how to go through a maze, other rats in different locations coming after them learn faster when going through the same maze.

Finally, morphic resonance would explain why our IQ levels are rising: we are learning from all the people before us who have taken the same quizzes.

Recall the idea of COEX (Systems of Condensed Experiences) we mentioned in Chapter Six (page 101)? COEX is a chain of associations of memories, with the earlier memories having the most impact. We can also use the idea of morphic resonance to explain COEX.

Because memories of events generating the same emotions are very similar to each other by vibration, they resonate with each other and become organized together. Other similar experiences involving the same emotions are drawn in through morphic resonance / LOA, causing repetitive patterns of experiences that we can see in our life.

The woman who keeps attracting abusive partners, the businessman who keeps attracting fraud, or the student who keeps experiencing betrayals by her friends — all these are patterns that these people draw to themselves by their COEX structures.

Brought to its logical conclusion, there is a memory surrounding every species of living thing that seems to influence each member of the species. Living beings that are more similar are more likely to draw from the same memories. Inheritance may then be not just a simple matter of genes but an effect of morphic resonance.[95]

This memory surrounding every living thing is named the *morphogenetic field*, the field effect created by morphic resonance. A morphogenetic field coordinates the functions of bodies and provides a 'template' that a healthy body should follow. A body is considered healthy when it is able to resonate with this template and unhealthy when it's not able to resonate with it.

Now let's look at the discovery of *biophotons* by Professor Fritz-Albert Popp, a German researcher in biophysics. His work provides another perspective of the morphic resonance mechanism.

Morphogenetic Field is also the Light Field That Surrounds All Living Things

Simply put, all living things emit light that cannot be seen by the naked eye but that can be measured by special equipment. This light comes from *biophotons*, weak electromagnetic photon emissions from living organisms.

In cells, it's the DNA that is responsible for the storage and emission of biophotons. In fact, DNA's spiral shape is ideal for light storage because through rhythmic contractions DNA can store and emit light. The DNA first stashes away the light it receives, but sends it back out if it receives too much.

Professor Fritz-Albert Popp directed a light at living cells and discovered that they would absorb the light before releasing it. An even bigger discovery was that healthy cells and diseased cells seem to emit different amounts of biophotons. Healthy cells seem to emit fewer biophotons while diseased cells seem to emit more biophotons.

Professor Popp found that the DNA of a living organism shed more light when it was subjected to stress. This also happened when a person was feeling negative emotions; this caused the cells in that person's body to lose their ability to create, send or receive coherent light. The more diseased the tissues become, the more incoherent their biophoton emissions become.

What does coherence mean? It means being structured.

Why is being structured important? Because having structure is how information can be passed on.

If a cell realizes that it is becoming dysfunctional, its DNA sends out coherent light to reorganize itself back to its healthy configuration. This light contains information for the cell to heal itself.

Over time, the overall amount of light stored in the body of a sick person will be significantly reduced compared to that of a healthy person.[96]

If we combine all the light emissions of all the cells in the body, we get a common bio-field surrounding the body.[97] People have called this by different names, with the most common being *aura*.

Another name for this bio-field is the morphogenetic field — yes, the same morphogenetic field we spoke about when discussing morphic resonance.

The Body, Particularly the DNA, Tunes to the Morphogenetic Field to Retrieve Memories

Based on all the information we have about morphogenetic fields, it seems clear that these fields hold all the information and memories of all the events that have ever happened to the person, including events which happened beyond the current life of this person (this is discussed in later chapters).[98]

Information enters the DNA through light from the environment; light is then sent out by the DNA via biophotons to organize the body. This process is the morphogenetic field in action.

To believe in something seemingly invisible like morphogenetic fields may be difficult, so let's look at a metaphor that may make it easier to relate to the idea: the television.

The television provides us with images that are beamed from a station. It's not the television that is creating the images; the images come from invisible electromagnetic fields sent out from the station.

These fields continue to exist whether or not the television is there to pick them up.

It is true that in order to pick up the signals, the television — with all its electronic components working properly — is necessary. Therefore, for an alien from space who is visiting Earth and sees the television for the first time, it's easy to think that it's the television that is creating the images it sees.

In fact, a fault in any of the electronic components of the television can affect the quality of the image displayed; this further reinforces the belief that the interaction of the components of the television is what is producing the images.

Similarly, morphogenetic fields are the invisible fields around us. The brain picks up the signals and produces the memories that we know. If our brain gets severely damaged, we may experience amnesia. We may therefore think the brain holds the memories, when it is actually the morphogenetic fields that are doing so.

To repeat: it is the morphogenetic fields that hold memories; the brain is merely a transmitter and receiver of these thoughts. In fact, I believe that it's the DNA in every cell of the body that is the actual transmitter and receiver of information, while the brain is the central processing unit that takes the memories from all parts of the body and gives us a holistic experience by combining these memories together.

(This would mean that life after death, which we looked at in Chapter Three when introducing NDEs [Near-Death Experiences, page 56], is possible. Even though there is no longer a physical body to receive the transmission (just like a broken television), the stream of consciousness of the person who died still exists as an invisible field, independent of a physical body. This stream of consciousness is the morphogenetic field.)

The morphogenetic field has been found to control all metabolic processes in the body, including the switching on and off of DNA, creation of enzymes, and breakdown of proteins into amino acids, amongst other important functions. Every disease always starts with a disturbance first in the morphogenetic field; this disturbance then filters down into the physical body.[99]

Genetic mutations are not programmed into the genes. To use our television analogy again, the mutation affects the body's 'tuning system' so that it is not able to receive certain information from the morphogenetic field surrounding it.

For example, fruit flies have been found to be born with legs in places where wings are supposed to be. Instead of saying that a fly's genes wrongly programmed legs onto the wings, it's probably more accurate to say that genetic mutations caused that part of the body to resonate with a different field: the field for legs instead of that for wings. As a result, the legs grew in the place that the wings were supposed to be.[100]

There is an original *perfect health blueprint* held as a memory in the morphogenetic field that the cells in our body resonate with in ideal conditions. Memories that hold an emotional charge, eg traumas, cause us to fall out of resonance with this original blueprint. Disturbances caused by traumas affect how much of the morphogenetic field we can access. In a bid to increase the flow of information to the rest of the body, more biophotons in the DNA of cells have to be emitted. Since we can now access less of the morphogenetic field, our biochemical and metabolic processes are affected. This reinforces our picture that trauma memories can create stress in the body that eventually leads to disease.

Summary

It's time to bring together all the different concepts relating to memories.

Firstly, we learned from the previous chapter that past traumas can sustain current illnesses. Regardless of how long ago they occurred, past traumas can continue to haunt us and make us sick by activating the stress response in our body that prevents our body from detoxing. There must therefore be some structure in the body for these memories, and indeed, there is.

We introduced the idea of cellular memories: that all cells in the body hold the memories of past events. At the micro-level in the cell, it is the DNA that is the physical storage for memories, but that's not the whole story. There is a morphogenetic field surrounding everyone that contains the cumulative memories of all the events that have ever happened to us as well as other beings very similar to us.

The DNA, cell and brain — going from the micro-level to the macro-level — are merely tuning devices that tap into this morphogenetic field. Memories are recorded in this field and can be retrieved as well. These memories are organized according to similarity and association and form a COEX chain, with the earliest memories having the greatest influence. Looking only at our current life, womb and birth memories have the most impact, followed by childhood memories and finally adult memories. These trauma memories continue to form an 'attractor field' that draws similar traumatic experiences to us repeatedly.

If our current life were the be-all and end-all of our experiences then this would be the conclusion of the book. But life is more complex than that. In the next four chapters, we venture into how our trauma memories may *not* be directly related to an experience from our current life.

We mentioned that morphogenetic fields may hold the cumulative memories of all species. We also mentioned DNA as the physical storage of these memories, so what is the role of the genes in DNA in disease formation? We have been led to believe that genes hold the key to disease. Is this really true? This topic is discussed in Chapter Eight when we discuss genes, both the conventional view and the reality.

In addition, if the memories (in the morphogenetic field) of species similar to us have some effect on our health, then the memories of human beings should affect our health even more, and the memories of people who were most similar to us — our ancestral line — should have the greatest impact on our health. This sets the stage for Chapter Nine: how traumas that affected our ancestors are also shaping our health.

In Chapter Ten, we explore how we could have lived multiple lives through the process of reincarnation and therefore how traumas in those lives could also be guiding the course of our health in our current life.

In Chapter Eleven, we look at the highly controversial topic of how entities or spirits could be hijacking our morphogenetic fields and causing our diseases.

EIGHT — Genes: It's Not Destiny!

The Human Genome Project Changed Our Idea of How Genes Work

2000 CE. President Bill Clinton, US President, is addressing the crowd at the White House as he hails the completion of the preliminary survey of the Human Genome Project. He believes this will revolutionize the way medicine works, and how most if not all diseases will be cured with this breakthrough.[101]

2001 CE. The Human Genome Project has been officially completed. It reveals that human beings are almost identical at the DNA level. In fact, not just humans but dolphins, rats, mice, dogs, chickens and even fish all have almost identical DNA.[102] As genes code for proteins, and there are 70,000 to 90,000 proteins in the human body, it was expected that there would be more than 90,000 genes responsible for the human genetic make-up. However, only around 23,000 genes were found (today, that number has shrunk to 19,000!). In fact, we have fewer genes than rice, which has 38,000 genes![103]

2009 CE. Twenty-seven of the best geneticists in the world — including Francis Collins, the former head of the Human Genome Project — published a paper in the prestigious journal, *Nature*, declaring that despite an expense of more than US$100 billion, they had found only a very limited genetic basis for human diseases. This problem is now known as the 'missing heritability problem'.[104]

The 'Missing Heritability Problem' Means That Genes Cannot Possibly Explain Disease

Given the height of the parents, a child's height can be predicted with an accuracy of up to 80-90 percent. Height must therefore be inherited.

When scientists looked for the genes that code for height, they found about fifty genes which determine whether a person is tall or short. In combination though, these genes account for only 5 percent of a height value. The missing 75-85 percent, which cannot be accounted for by 'height genes', baffles scientists.[105]

Similarly, 'schizophrenia genes' are unable to account for schizophrenia, 'cancer genes' do not account for cancer, and 'diabetes genes' cannot account for Type 2 diabetes. The same is true with many other complex diseases.

In a characteristic move, scientists now want to increase sample sizes, hoping that increasing the number of people tested in a trial may change the trial outcomes. Could scientists once again be ignoring the fact that they may have made certain fundamental assumptions about genes that are in error?

The main assumption here can be traced back to 1953. When Sir Francis Crick revealed the double-helix structure of the DNA, he also proposed the idea, known in molecular biology as the Central Dogma, that genes are responsible for all our characteristics.[106] This paradigm is so entrenched in the ideology of molecular biologists that any data that does not fit this theory of genetic determinism is automatically dismissed!

So are genes really what they are made out to be: unalterable and the cause of all disease?

Our DNA is made up of 3 percent Genes and 97 percent *Junk DNA*

When your father's sperm first met your mother's egg, the first cell of what would eventually become you was created. In the nucleus of this first cell, a DNA molecule — shaped like a coiled double helix — was formed comprising 23 chromosomes from your father and 23 chromosomes from your mother for a total of 46 chromosomes. Each of these 23 pairs of chromosomes may contain anywhere from hundreds to thousands of genes.

This first cell would eventually divide and form all the organs in your body, from your brain to your bones. Therefore, your DNA is found in the nucleus of almost every cell of your body, and is virtually identical in every cell. The sum total of your DNA is known as your *genome*.[107] Your genome is made up of 3.1 billion amino-acid base pairs.[108]

Your DNA can be likened to a book about you: it contains all the information needed to build and maintain your body. Your amino-acid base pairs can be likened to the letters of the alphabet in this book.

The fundamental building blocks of your body, however, are not DNA but proteins. Proteins are used for all cellular functions, including producing enzymes, digesting our food, and creating an appropriate immune response if you are exposed to toxins.[109] We can think of DNA as containing the blueprint used to construct proteins. The DNA is first 'read'. A protein is then made based on the specifications provided in that part of the DNA.

Scientists have a naming convention:

- 'Genes' are the parts of our DNA that code for proteins;
- 'Junk DNA' is the parts of our DNA that do not code for proteins.

Out of our entire DNA, only an astonishingly low figure of 3 percent code for proteins.[110] When this was discovered, scientists were shocked that the number of genes was fewer than the number of proteins we make: it had been intuitively assumed that we'd have one gene for each type of protein we have in the body.

The remaining 97 percent of our DNA — the vast majority of our DNA — is known as 'junk DNA' simply because of the belief that if it didn't code for anything material like proteins, there couldn't possibly be anything useful about it.[111]

Junk DNA Determines the Regulation of Genes and is the Source of Epigenetics

New research into junk DNA is showing that it's not as useless as believed.

For example, over a million unique structures of 'jumping DNA' have been found in junk DNA. This jumping DNA is capable of breaking loose and settling down elsewhere on the DNA strand, thereby rewriting the DNA code. [112] In other words, the primary structure of DNA can change.

Medical science has traditionally believed that our lives are predetermined by our genetic material. But if our DNA can change all the time (and now we know it can), then what we have been led to believe — that our genes are our destiny — may not be true after all.

8 - Genes: It's Not Destiny!

Does simply having the genes to construct a certain protein mean that this protein will be built in a perfect chain of events? The answer is 'No'.

Your gene represents only potential; only when the DNA is 'read' and the protein created do we move from potential (like a planner's blueprint) to expression (like a finished building). The fact is that problems can arise in the process from blueprint to building.

Firstly, perhaps there is a mutation in some genes — for an analogy, think of a misspelling in a book — which would mean that the final version of the protein created would have a flaw. Sometimes, this may not be a big deal. At other times, this can be deadly if the protein in question serves a vital purpose in the body.

Secondly, perhaps some part of the DNA cannot be read — again, an analogy would be a piece of bubble gum between two pages of a book, preventing those two pages from being read — meaning that the protein coded by that portion of the DNA cannot be constructed. This happens because certain enzymes may stimulate a section of the DNA to wrap itself tightly so that section cannot be read. (Other enzymes can stimulate it to relax and uncoil itself.)

A gene is said to be 'switched on' when the DNA is relaxed and can be read *(transcribed)*, and 'switched off' when the DNA helix is coiled and cannot be read. [113] (The scientific terms for these phenomena are *DNA methylation* and *DNA acetylation*. See figure next page.)

Junk DNA serves as a regulation mechanism for genes: it switches genes on and off appropriately in order to control how much of each protein is to be produced and when. Junk DNA appears to serve as the contractor who organizes the building materials (genes) to ensure that the building parts (proteins) are constructed optimally.

Epigenetics

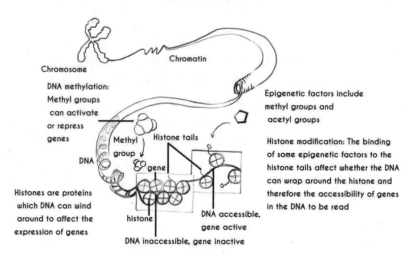

Figure 8: Epigenetics in Action

Genetic expression appears to be all about awaiting a signal to start the process of protein creation. Scientists have for the longest time focused on the process of how proteins are created, but not on what signals could be responsible for triggering this process. Both environmental influences — our diet, exposure to toxins — and emotions — the emotions our ancestors felt, and the emotions we experienced in our childhood — can serve as these signals.[114]

These signals are picked up from the morphogenetic field (see Chapter Seven, page 124) that stores all our memories. These signals then affect our 'jumping DNA', those sections of DNA that can move around, thus changing the structure of our DNA.

The science of *epigenetics* — the study of mechanisms that switch genes on or off — is now thought to hold the key to many of the mysteries of life. Epigenetics means 'above the genes': influences on genetic expression that occur outside the gene itself. The crux of epigenetics is the 'switching on' and 'switching off' of genes.

An analogy, again from the book world, is: which pages of the book (DNA) are being read will determine what is to be produced (proteins) at any given time.

Recall that we'd mentioned a missing heritability problem (page 131), the fact that scientists had not been able to find a clear link between genes and disease. Initial studies are showing that epigenetics can have a crucial impact on diseases such as autism, diabetes, multiple sclerosis, etc.[115] The epigenetics link is further explored in Chapter Nine.

DNA May Actually Be a Wave of Information

Dr. Peter Gariaev, PhD, is a Russian scientist who is now known as a pioneer in the field of *wave genetics*, the science of using fields and waves to influence DNA.

In an experiment one day, he placed a sample of DNA inside a quartz container and zapped it with a mild laser. Using sensitive equipment that could detect even single photons of light, Dr. Gariaev observed that the DNA strand absorbed all the photons of light, storing them in a corkscrew-shaped spiral.

When the experiment concluded, Dr. Gariaev packed the container and DNA away but discovered, to his great surprise, that the light continued to spiral along in the spot where the DNA had been placed. This 'DNA image' lasted for thirty full days and is now known as the 'DNA Phantom Effect'. There is only one possible meaning of this finding: there is an energetic double to the physical DNA.[116]

Today, scientists are fervently looking for a way to use gene therapy to heal all kinds of diseases. This is resource-intensive and time-consuming work because, for every trial, the relevant gene — a microscopic structure — has to be isolated and physically manipulated.

Dr. Gariaev reasoned that if physical DNA has an energetic double, DNA can actually be thought of as a wave that contains information. If this was true, it would be much simpler to modify the information in DNA by using laser light to transmit the new information into the DNA. A laser is most appropriate as it provides extremely organized light, making it ideal for carrying information.

If new information, carried via the medium of laser light, could change DNA, this could create just the kind of healing effects that scientists, currently physically tinkering with genes using gene therapy, were hoping to achieve.

In a series of experiments, Dr. Gariaev was able to show that his hypothesis was on the right track. For example, he found some seeds, at the site of the disused Chernobyl nuclear reactor, which had died from radiation poisoning. He shone a low-intensity (non-burning) laser light though healthy seeds from the same kind of plant into these dead seeds. The dead seeds completely healed and grew into healthy adult plants.[117]

Dr. Gariaev performed a similar experiment, this time on animals. He injected into rats a lethal dose of a toxin called alloxan that would destroy their pancreas and cause them to die from diabetes type 1 within four to six days. He then shone a laser beam through the pancreas and spleen of a healthy rat into the poisoned rats. About 90 percent of the rats recovered completely, with a regenerated pancreas and eventually normalized blood sugar levels, within 12 days. Even more amazingly, he could obtain the exact same results when transmitting the beam from twenty kilometers away![118]

To treat an elderly woman for diabetes, Dr. Gariaev attempted to regenerate her pancreas by energizing her ten-year-old grandson's blood and beaming it into her using healing frequencies. According to his hypothesis, a child's DNA has an energy signature similar to that of the DNA of his parents and grandparents, albeit in a younger and healthier configuration. Dr. Gariaev used a specially modified wide-spectrum red laser for this treatment.

Unexpectedly, the elderly woman, who had only one tooth left, started feeling pain and swelling in her jaw. Out grew three new wisdom teeth! We have been taught in elementary biology that a person has only two sets of teeth, one set as children and another set that develops in adulthood. This elderly woman had had both these sets of teeth, yet by being subjected to light carrying a healthy 'energy signature' had somehow managed to grow a third, partial set of teeth![119]

Dr. Gariaev now believes, based on his mind-boggling findings, that DNA is first and foremost an energetic structure that then organizes the physical DNA structure.

This, of course, is completely contrary to the position of many of his contemporaries. It is no surprise then that his ideas are too radical for them to accept and that he has been shunned by his contemporaries, even though his findings have been backed up by hard experimental evidence.

If DNA is indeed first an information wave — that then manifests as a physical DNA structure — and all living creatures have very similar DNA (see the beginning of this Chapter), could changing the information in the DNA using wave genetics even lead to the creation of different species of plants and animals?

New Species Can Be Created by Manipulating DNA Using Laser

Dr. Gariaev shone a green, non-burning laser through salamander eggs, and then redirected the laser into frog eggs. The frog eggs were completely transformed into salamander eggs, and normal salamanders hatched. These salamanders were completely healthy; in time, they too produced normal, healthy salamander offspring.[120]

At this point, you may be wondering if anyone else was able to replicate Dr. Gariaev's results. After all, reproducibility or replication is one of the principles of the scientific method.

In 1993, Korean scientist Dr. Dzang Kangeng managed to produce a chicken-duck hybrid bird by transferring the genetic code of a duck into a hen using an energy wave. He zapped the duck with a high-frequency electrostatic generator, and directed the energy into another room where a pregnant hen was placed for five days.

The creatures that subsequently hatched from the hen's eggs had a flat beak, longer neck and larger internal organs — all features characteristic of ducks. They were also significantly heavier than the average chicken. The experiment was repeated with 500 eggs; of these, 480 hatched, and 384 of the 480 chicks were chicken-duck hybrids. The hybrid birds were able to breed with each other, and their offspring were hybrids just like them.[121]

Ciba-Geigy, a chemical company, patented a process in 1989 where they were able to produce new and original species of plants and animals merely by running a weak current through seeds or eggs placed between two metal plates. They successfully created a formerly extinct species of fern with forty-one chromosomes rather than the normal thirty-six. Similarly, they produced an older version of wheat that could be harvested within four to eight weeks instead of the normal seven months. By repeating the process on trout eggs, they were able to create a new species of trout that was stronger and more disease-resistant.[122]

DNA Draws Information from Morphogenetic Fields to Determine Which Form It Should Take

Based on all these examples, here is my hypothesis.

There seems to be a universal DNA — one that is the same for all living species — but the way it is structured determines what species it expresses. DNA is first an energetic structure; this DNA can be changed by transmitting new information using a laser light. Whether we become a human, an animal or a plant depends on how our DNA taps into the field of information that surrounds us. These fields must be the morphogenetic fields we first mention in Chapter 7 (page 124).

All living things thus tap into these morphogenetic fields, drawing the accumulated memories of their particular species to structure themselves. The morphogenetic field they tap into is the field they are most attuned to, depending on their vibration (frequency). We have labelled these, based broadly on their expression, as human, animal or plant.

The DNA in our cells is merely a 'tuning device' to access the morphogenetic field that surrounds all of us. The information in this field influences our junk DNA to switch genes on and off appropriately, producing the appropriate proteins and enzymes required by each particular species of living things.

Mainstream science, focusing more on the physical makeup of DNA in terms of genes, instead of the morphogenetic field which the DNA picks up information from to order the physical body, actually has it all mixed up.

Summary

So what are the implications of these findings?

First of all, these findings show that what we have learnt from mainstream thinking about genes is very different from what new research into the area is telling us. Genes are traditionally believed to control every one of our attributes: influence our birth; determine when we die; and govern the kinds of illnesses we suffer from between birth and death.

However, the latest research from epigenetics and junk DNA shows otherwise: genes are not everything. Only around 3 percent of our DNA is genes; the remaining 97 percent, misclassified as 'junk DNA', determines how these genes get expressed. The latter therefore seems more critical in determining our physical characteristics.

Secondly, we are taught to think that genes are unchangeable: we have to live with what we are born with. I hope you can see by now that if a laser light can change a frog's egg to produce a salamander, or regenerate certain organs, then it's definitely possible that genes, or the way they are expressed, could be altered too.

Thirdly, our genes and our DNA are not just physical structures; there is an energetic equivalent of DNA that can be manipulated to perform healing or even to produce new species never before seen.

Finally, if our DNA is merely tapping into the morphogenetic field that surrounds the body in order to organize the body then our obsession with genes is misguided. Instead, if morphogenetic fields are indeed the cumulative sum of all memories, then these memories must be affecting our health, as Chapter Six (pages 102 to 105) argues.

Chapter Six shows us that our womb, birth and childhood memories seem to play a major part in how we contract disease later on in life; the exact mechanism for this is detailed in Chapter Seven. We hypothesized that the earlier the memory, the more strongly it influences us.

It's now time to explore the memories we have that come from even before our current life. In the next chapter, we explore *ancestral traumas* or *trans-generational traumas* — the traumas of our ancestors — and how they can still be affecting us even when our ancestors are no longer physically around.

NINE — Epigenetics: Taking on Your Ancestors Fate

The Dutch Famine Illustrates How Lack of Food in One Generation Can Affect the Health of the Next Two Generations

It was the winter of 1944. The tide of World War II had shifted against the Nazis, but the Netherlands was still occupied.

It had been one of the harshest winters ever, and food was extremely scarce. At one point, the Dutch had had to resort to eating grass and tulip bulbs to survive. Daily calorie intake had plunged to a shocking 30 per cent of normal. By May 1945, when food supplies were finally restored, more than 20,000 people had died. The event is known as the Dutch Famine.

Years passed. The natural inclination would be to think that the people who survived that period would move on and life would return to normal. That inclination would be wrong. A study done on a group of the survivors is eye opening.

The study found that a mother who had been malnourished in the first three months of gestation would produce a baby that came out seemingly perfectly healthy at birth but that would end up much more likely to be obese in adulthood. Daughters born to these mothers had twice the rate of schizophrenia compared to the norm.

The tragic but expected effects of war, you say. There was more.

Remarkably, these effects were replicated in the *grandchildren* of the survivors. Something traumatic that had happened to one generation of the population came to have an impact on two later generations (and possibly additional ones)!

Apparently, epigenetic changes to several genes, responsible for growth and development, had taken place. [123] In conventional biology, this should not and could not happen: changes outside genes could not possibly survive transmission to the next generation. The effects of famine on one generation could not have passed on to the next generation. [124]

Lamarck was Right in Saying that Environmental Factors Can Affect the Expression of Genes and be inherited by Subsequent Generations

To understand why conventional biological science holds this belief, we have to look at two individuals who had radically different theories about how living things evolve. The first scientist is someone that everyone has heard of: Charles Darwin. The second scientist is Jean Baptiste Lamarck, whom few people have heard of.

Charles Darwin is of course the Father of Evolution, the discoverer of the *theory of natural selection* – the process, according to current mainstream thought, by which living things evolve. This theory is based on three fundamental assumptions:

1. Firstly, all organisms descend from a common ancestor;
2. Secondly, species evolve through random mutations which do not derive from the environment; and
3. Thirdly, that these mutations pass on to subsequent generations only if they give the animals with these

mutations a survival advantage over those that do not have these mutations.

Evolution is ultimately seen as a process in which the strongest triumph over the weakest — with the difference between these two groups being only a matter of random mutations.[125]

Lamarck believed in a different kind of evolution, a process known as 'inheritance of acquired characteristics'. He believed that evolution in a living thing, say an animal, happens through a cooperative effort between the animal and its environment. If an animal is exposed to a certain environment, it would acquire certain characteristics during its lifetime in response to stresses in the environment. These characteristics could then be passed on to its offspring.[126]

In his lifetime, Lamarck's theory was denounced; he eventually died penniless. Yet results from the Dutch Famine prove that Lamarck was not wrong after all. An environmental effect — a lack of food — caused changes in the way genes responsible for growth and development were expressed, changes that were subsequently passed down to at least two generations.

Epigenetics Shows How Two Genetically Identical Persons Can Have Different Fates Depending on Whether Certain Genes are Switched On or Off

This idea that environmental factors could alter genetic coding, as shown in the Dutch Famine, has now been given a name: *epigenetics*. The related word *epigenome* means a record of chemical changes to the DNA during our lifetime. Epigenetics is the hot new buzzword in medicine, for a very good reason: all kinds of diseases like cancer, diabetes and coronary heart disease have now been found to be associated with it.

To understand epigenetics a little more and contrast it with genetics, let's look at a specific example.

Let's say we have a pair of identical twins. Identical twins have the exact same genome, the complete set of genes or genetic material. So if diseases were linked to genes only, you would expect identical twins to be afflicted with the same kinds of diseases. Yet if one identical twin has schizophrenia, there is only a 50 percent chance that the other twin would have the same condition. Although this is significantly higher than the 1 percent risk that a person from the general population has of getting schizophrenia, it is also much smaller than the 100 percent we would expect if genes alone fully predicted disease.[127]

Hence, any difference between two genetically identical individuals must be traceable to epigenetics. Somehow, there have been modifications, a result of environmental influences, affecting which genes are now switched on or switched off, but the genes themselves have not been changed. (Recall that in the body, the switching on and off of genes is executed by certain enzymes. See Chapter Eight, page 135 for details.)

All Traumas Create Epigenetic Effects

In epigenetics, we also see the memory mechanism at work. An event in the environment triggers a change in the way genes express, and the biological effect on the body continues to last long after the event is over.

Remember how we mentioned that womb, birth and childhood traumas could trigger disease years after the initial event (the discussion begins Chapter Six, page 102)? Apparently, all these traumas must have created an epigenetic effect when they happened.

This has been demonstrated in mouse studies. For example, mice were separated from their mother at birth. Remember the hypothalamus-pituitary-gland-adrenals axis (HPA Axis), connected to the stress response, that we mentioned in Chapter Four (page 71)? Arginine vasopressin is secreted by the hypothalamus to stimulate secretion from the pituitary gland. In mice that are separated from their mother, the arginine vasopressin gene becomes more expressed, causing a greater stress response.

By the end of the tenth day of birth, this expression of genes has become 'fixed'. Stress hormones continue to be pumped out and the mice continue to feel highly stressed, even if they are subsequently returned to their mothers. The triggering event — being separated from the mother — has caused a permanent rewiring of their gene expression.[128]

The results of the above study show that something that happens early in current life can cause an epigenetic effect later in life. The Dutch Famine shows that this epigenetic effect can affect subsequent generations.

So what happens if this epigenetic effect is undone? How can that change the health of a person?

When an Epigenetic Effect is Undone, Supposedly Incurable Diseases can be Reversed

In Rett's Syndrome, a rare disease that is almost exclusively found in girls, one of the most damaging symptoms is mental retardation. It involves a gene known as the Mecp2 gene. The general view on mental retardation is that it is incurable and non-reversible, yet a study by Adrian Bird, Ph.D., shows that it's possible to reverse it in mice if the epigenetic effect is undone.

Bird started by creating a cloned strain of mice and inactivating the Mecp2 gene, effectively brain damaging the mice. However, he also engineered things such that the mice carried a normal copy of the Mecp2 gene, with the normal copy 'switched off'.

The mice that were subsequently born exhibited symptoms very similar to Rett's syndrome in humans. They hardly moved about and wouldn't explore anything when placed in a box, unlike normal curious mice.

Then, using a chemical, the normal copy of the Mecp2 gene in the mice was switched on. The transformation was astonishing. The mice that had earlier shown all the symptoms of mental retardation began scurrying around, just like normal mice.

This suggests that perhaps everything needed to make the brain functional is already there in the brain's makeup; the appropriate genes just need to be switched on — and, as already mentioned, the switching on and off of genes is just epigenetics at work. If these kinds of results can happen to mice, they can happen to humans.[129]

The effects of epigenetic are not just the domain of scientists. Psychotherapists have independently found a similar phenomenon — trans-generational effects — in their clinical work with clients.

'Invisible Loyalty' Explains Why a Trauma from an Ancestor Can Continue to Affect Us

Anne Ancelin Schutzenberger was one of the pioneers of trans-generational psychotherapy. She became interested in this work when she realized, through a chance conversation with her daughter, that she was the only surviving member of two siblings. Improbably, her husband was also the only surviving member of two siblings, and her daughter was the only surviving member of two children! Even more bizarrely, all the people who had passed away in her family had died from car accidents![130]

I have my own uncanny family story. On one occasion my father was talking about his younger brother; from the look in his eyes, I could see the love he had had for him. Unfortunately, this brother fell ill and died, around one year of age, during the Second World War (1939-1945).

My father then shared how my elder brother, his first son, had contracted a very high fever and almost died — at age one. Although my father mentioned both incidents together, he didn't then understand the implications of linking the two stories as he had done, though the 'coincidence' of my elder brother almost following in the footsteps of my father's younger brother were immediately apparent to me.

Anne had a term for this phenomenon: *invisible loyalties.*[131] Again and again, she found cases of descendants unconsciously paying off 'debts' from the past to their ancestors.

It appears we are doomed to repeat moments of sorrow, injustice, separation and death, whatever our ancestors experienced, unless the link is broken.

Young children have a strong impulse to love their parents. I remember that, when I was young and living with my parents who, with three children in tow, were struggling to make ends meet, I made a vow: "Let me take on my parents' suffering and make their burdens lighter". This natural impulse to love and belong causes us to take on the pain of our parents as if they were our own, not knowing that in the process, no one actually gains.[132]

When we make a decision to take on the misery of our parents, we either become exactly like them (including taking on their flaws), or we absorb their anguish to an extent that ensures we never become more than them.

This often shows up in people who find that no matter how hard they work they cannot progress. To thrive would be to 'betray' their parents. After all, who are they to be successful when their parents are stuck in a rut or in misery?

Then there is often a member of the family who becomes what we called the 'fixer'. The fixer takes on the role of counseling, healing and helping other family members. She may even choose the path of staying single to take care of her aging parents. In many people's books, she plays the role of a hero.

At the other end is the black sheep of the family. This person — typically an alcoholic, a compulsive gambler or a womanizer — conventionally is the epitome of badness and immorality. Yet perhaps this person is the way he is because he is trying to take on the afflictions of an ancestor and lighten the family load for the rest of us.

Somewhere between these two extremes we may find the martyr: someone who becomes ill to alleviate the wrongdoings of her ancestors.

Fixer, black sheep and martyr: are the roles really that straightforward? The common element in these seemingly very different roles is the impulse to love and take on the hurt of ancestors. In the world of the invisible, good and bad may not be so clear-cut.

So what are some common traumas that could have affected our ancestors, and, through the invisible links of loyalty, us?

A Child Given Away Would Have to Be Atoned For By Someone Else in the Family

My maternal uncle is mentally unstable. The problem started in university: he met and fell in love with a girl but the relationship met with huge opposition from his father. Finally, my uncle split with the girl but he was never the same again.

It is easy to assign blame for my uncle's condition on this one incident. However, trace the history of my mother's family and we find the roots of his mental illness appearing long before he was born.

My uncle was the eighth child of my maternal grandparents. The first seven were all girls; six of them — all of them except my mother — were given away for adoption by my grandparents. Why would a family give away six of its children?

My maternal aunts were born in an age and culture when boys were prized more than girls. My grandfather was a chauvinist steeped in the belief that boys would carry on the family line while females would only become a burden. In fact, he gave my mother a Chinese name meaning "Seventh Slave"; throughout her life, she struggled with a need to do everything for everyone else, in an unconscious bid to earn the fatherly love that she never got.

According to the invisible-loyalty principle, the debt of a person given away by the family would have to be atoned for by someone else in the family.[133] It is ironic that, through my uncle, my grandfather managed to get the male heir to the family line that he so desperately sought, but that my uncle then, by becoming mentally ill, took on the guilt of my grandfather for giving away six of his daughters.

This also applies to adopters, the family that accepts a child belonging to another family. Sometimes, the family that adopts a child feels an unconscious guilt as if they have 'stolen a child' from another family.[134]

Someone in the Family May End Up Representing a Sibling Who Died in a Miscarriage or Abortion

At the age of 3, Deyaan began to flap his hands, grind his teeth and walk aimlessly from cabinet to cabinet. He stopped speaking and started ignoring family and relatives. His worried parents, suspecting he had autism, brought him to see me.

During a session, I found out that his parents had aborted a child just before it was to be born. At the time the parents hadn't wanted children and had jointly decided to go for an abortion.

However, at the session, looking at the grief expressed by the mother when she faced her feelings about the decision, I could see that she had buried her feelings about it.

When the mother was finally able to acknowledge the abortion and seek forgiveness from her aborted child, there was an amazing transformation in Deyaan. His behavior rapidly improved and he started speaking.

Children who have died young, or been miscarried, aborted or stillborn, can leave an indelible print on the family.[135] Many parents usually repress their grief; this child becomes a secret no one talks about.

I have found a surprising number of cases of autistic children born into a family where a child has been lost. There may be a gap of a generation or two, ie the child lost may be a sibling of the parents or even the grandparents. For example, the father of another autistic child had lost his younger sister when she drowned in a well.

I call this phenomenon the 'lost child phenomenon': a child had been lost in the family (from a miscarriage, stillbirth, abortion or childhood accident); when another child was born in the 'family' (perhaps a later generation), the autistic child had an invisible bond of loyalty to that lost child, in effect also becoming 'lost' to the family.

The fact of a lost child may have been long forgotten or even lost as new generations of the family arose; no one in the current generation might even be aware of it.

There is another phenomenon known as the 'vanishing twin phenomenon'. In brief, this is a situation where there had originally been twins *in-utero* (before birth), but somewhere during gestation one of the twins died and was reabsorbed by the surviving twin.

When the child was born, it would naturally be assumed that there had always been only one child in the womb; the child who had died, never being discovered, would never be acknowledged. One out of every eight pregnancies is believed to involve the vanishing twin phenomenon; in most cases, obviously, there is no reason even to expect it.[136]

I myself had a vanishing twin who was somehow discovered (during a process which will be covered in my second book, *Reversing the Disease Code*).

The vanishing-twin phenomenon manifests as 'survivor guilt': the surviving twin frequently sabotages his success because he feels guilty for having lived when his twin died. Patterns such as huge financial losses, relationship breakups, alcohol abuse, etc, are common scenarios for the surviving twin. Many of the survivors also grow up with suicidal thoughts and depression because they have an unconscious drive to follow their twin.[137]

In Japan there is a ritual for children who die before or shortly after birth. The child is known as *mizuko* ('unseeing child') and this ritual is called *mizuki kuyo*. It involves an offering to Jizo, a *bodhisattva* (a Sanskrit term meaning a person who is able to attain *nirvana* but delays doing so out of compassion for suffering beings) who protects children, requesting the mizuko to move into the spiritual world and seek rebirth.[138]

Rituals aside, the important thing seems to be to acknowledge, respect and honor the lost child and grant her a place of residence in the heart of her parents.

Sudden Deaths Can Cause another Person to Follow In the Footsteps

Shakeela had relentless suicidal thoughts; they kept coming up despite her repeated attempts to shut them out. She had already slashed her wrists a few times but never cut really deep. She had been diagnosed with psychosis; her father, who had schizophrenia, had committed suicide a few years ago. In another case, Lena, who suffered from chronic fatigue, had a brother who had died in an accident in the army.

In both these cases, one or more surviving members of the family were drawn by an invisible bond of loyalty to follow in the footsteps of a family member who had died. This attraction could manifest itself consciously (in the case of Shakeela, through repeated attempts at suicide) or unconsciously (in Lena's case, through a chronic illness that might eventually become so debilitating that it would lead to death).

In fact, sudden death is linked to *disassociation* with our ancestors. It's a way of attracting attention to the fact that something has gone wrong in the family and the problem needs to be redressed. When these are addressed properly (usually by shamans, of the ancient traditions, performing the rituals developed specifically for the purpose), the descendants receive the blessings of their ancestors, bringing forth health, prosperity and joy.

One ritual at death performed for this very purpose — invoking the blessings of their ancestors — is done by the Native Americans (of North and South America), who build an altar and tend to it for a year, before taking it apart and saying prayers to release the departed soul.[139]

Now let's look at what happens when we don't accept a member of the family, by cutting off or breaking ties with them.[140]

Isolating, or Causing Injustice to, a Member of the Family Can Cause Disease to Descendants

Derrick was suffering from severe depression and anxiety. His father had died from lung cancer two years ago. Before his father passed away, they had made a trip to China.

Derrick's father had never seen his own mother (Derrick's grandmother). When Derrick's father was still very young, Derrick's grandfather had abandoned his wife in China and told her, "Just forget about me and marry someone else".

Derrick's grandmother replied, "No, since I have married into this family, I will die a member of this family".

Derrick's grandfather brought Derrick's father to Singapore and re-married. The grandmother in China was so grieved and cried so much that she went blind. Years passed.

On the trip to China, Derrick's father managed to locate the mother he had never seen.

Derrick still remembers the scene of their reunion. His grandmother slowly traced the face of her son, and said with much regret, "Why did you take so long to come back and see me?"

When it came time to leave, Derrick's father gave money to the relatives and asked them to take care of his mother for him. Derrick's grandmother was reluctant to let them go. "I have not been with you for long, and you are all going so quickly."

Not long after Derrick and his father returned to Singapore, they received news that Derrick's grandmother had died. Within a year, Derrick's father also passed away from lung cancer. (Lung cancer, if you recall from Chapter Five, page 107, is about repressed grief.)

Derrick can trace his own symptoms to the fact that his grandmother was isolated and not properly acknowledged, within the family, for her position as the first wife of his grandfather.

Finally, let's look at the phenomenon known as 'historical unresolved grief'.[141]

Historical Unresolved Grief is the Phenomenon of Perpetrators and Victims in a Larger Historical Context

From 1975-1979, a period when a communist regime known as the Khmer Rouge regime ruled Kampuchea (formerly Cambodia), 1.7 to 2.5 million people out of a 1975 population of about 8 million, died from execution, disease and starvation across a number of locations in Kampuchea known as the 'Killing Fields'. It is one of the worst genocides ever recorded in human history.

In Australia, during the period 1905 to 1969 and perhaps even later, mixed-race children of Australian Aboriginal and Torres Strait Islander descent were forcibly taken away from their families by the Australian Federal and State governments. This group of people is now known as the 'Stolen Generations'.

If our theories about trans-generational traumas are true, the events of the 'Killing Fields' era and the 'Stolen Generations' should have deep trans-generational effects on the descendants, the Kampucheans and Aborigines alive today. As these events happened relatively recently, the effects are not likely to be obvious yet.

However, researchers have already documented evidence of this epigenetic effect from other historical events; the effect has been termed 'historical unresolved grief'. For example, high rates of alcoholism, suicide and violence are found in Native Americans, living on the reservations, whose ancestors were violently affected by the colonization of their lands by European settlers.

The children of the survivors of the Nazi concentration and extermination camps — built during the Second World War with the purpose of demoralizing, dehumanizing or mass-murdering Jews, communists, socialists, Jehovah's Witnesses, homosexuals, gypsies and other 'unwanted' people or 'enemies of the state' — have been found to have higher stress levels, a fact that cannot possibly be explained by current-life traumas.[142]

Wars during which people died; genocides during which people were traumatized or suffered the loss of dearly loved ones; colonization or the slave trade during which the colonized and slaves endured death, extreme punishment and the taking away of children and land by the colonizers ... all these events sent colossal shock waves into the morphogenetic fields that surrounds all of us.

Modern Society Has Focused on the Nuclear Family over the Extended Family

Our modern society has idealized the concept of the nuclear family, so much so that many of us have lost touch with our extended family, a term that in the past included the dead as much as the living.

Many traditional cultures place a great deal of importance on making right the wrongs or injustices experienced by ancestors. On the other hand, we 'modern people' belittle these practices because we have no knowledge or understanding of why they are so important. Even when the hidden dynamics of these historical events affect our life, relationships, work and health, we fail to see, or understand the significance of, these connections to our past.

We don't live life purely as individuals, with no links to the past. As the morphogenetic fields show, individuals are linked to the cumulative memories of those who are similar to us. We can liken this to a 'family soul', a broader information field that includes all individuals, past and present, in the extended family.

Just like we can individually repress our feelings and cause illness in our own body, anyone in the extended family who has been 'pushed out of sight' can similarly cause a dysfunction in the family soul. This injustice would then have to be visited on another member of the family soul to redress this imbalance. Since morphogenetic fields go beyond space and time, the veil of death does not correct this imbalance. To restore these unrecognized ancestors to the family tree makes the family soul whole again, and allows everyone who is part of the family soul to attain peace.

Does this mean that once something has happened within a family line — say, to an earlier generation of the line — it will continue to trouble that family line for all remaining generations to come? How long can this epigenetic effect last?

The Effects of the Ancestral / Trans-Generational Traumas Seem to Rebalance Naturally in Three or Four Generations

Francis Hitching, a British author, writes of experiments on fruit flies in which he all the information in the DNA used to build the eyes was eliminated. As a result, new fruit flies were born blind. Five generations later, the fruit flies' eyes became normal again as if the DNA had never been lost.[143]

The Iroquois Confederacy, a group of Native Americans living in the northeastern part of the US, believed that any act done today would be felt by the next seven generations.[144] Even the Bible has its take on this issue: "The Lord is slow to anger and abounding in steadfast love, forgiving iniquity and transgression, but he will by no means clear the guilty, visiting the iniquity of the fathers on the children, to the third and the fourth generation".[145]

In my practice, I have found that this rebalancing of the family soul seems to take between three to four generations, on average.

Summary

The new field of epigenetics shows that the effects of traumas that affected one generation can be passed to subsequent generations. This proves that Lamarck (page 147) was right: organisms adapt based on stress from the environment and this can be inherited by subsequent generations. Epigenetics determines which genes are switched on and which are switched off, so it's not just the genes themselves that are important; we also have to look at the regulation of those genes.

Epigenetics has a memory mechanism: a trauma from the past can permanently switch on or switch off a gene, even in future generations. Hence, all traumas must have an epigenetics effect. It sounds plausible then that if the epigenetics effect can be altered we can radically change the expression of disease, even those that are considered incurable today.

What caused these epigenetic changes? The causes have to do with trans-generational traumas: traumas that affected our ancestors that then had a carry-over effect on us, their descendants. This is explained by the invisible-loyalties principle: within a family line, a descendant of a suffering ancestor would carry the fate of this ancestor out of unconscious loyalty towards the forebear.

An apt metaphor is the family soul. Any imbalance in the family soul has to be 'evened out' by someone else in the family. Imbalances include the giving up of children to other families or taking in of children from other families; 'unnatural' deaths of children such as abortions and miscarriages; sudden traumatic deaths; deaths due to wars, genocides and other conflicts; separation of family members, whether by choice (through cutting ties with someone) or by force (the Stolen Generation in the case of the Australian Aborigines).

From a holistic perspective, disease arises from a wider imbalance in the family and community from which we come. These imbalances are imprinted on the morphogenetic field as traumas coming from another generation. We extend this argument further in Chapter Fifteen when we get into even bigger systems. Before we come to that, however, we look at the controversial idea of multiple lives, and how traumas from past lives can have a bearing on our present life.

TEN — Past Lives: You have Lived Before

Well-Documented Studies Suggest Reincarnation Exists

Kendra Carter from Florida, United States, was a little girl barely five years of age when she went for her first lesson with a swimming coach named Ginger. Right from the start, Kendra took to Ginger; when Ginger had to cancel a lesson three weeks later, Kendra was inconsolable, and didn't recover until her swimming classes resumed.

A few weeks into the swimming lessons, Kendra mentioned that she was the little baby Ginger had lost about 14 years ago. She was able to describe vividly the scene of the abortion. Kendra's mother checked and discovered that Ginger had in fact had an abortion nine years before Kendra was born.

At some point, there was a falling out between Kendra's mother and Ginger. When Ginger refused to meet Kendra, Kendra didn't speak for almost five months. When Kendra finally met Ginger again, she spoke for the first time in five months and said that she loved Ginger.[146]

How was it that a little girl not yet five could describe abortion to the detail she had? Why would she claim that she was someone else's lost child, from an abortion that had happened years before she was born? Why would she demonstrate so much affection and attachment to Ginger? Furthermore, there is rich irony in Kendra's case: Kendra's mother belonged to a conservative Christian church, and the idea of reincarnation was a complete no-no.

Let's look at another phenomenon: cases of children born with birthmarks and features identical to that of people who had died before these children were born. Take the case of Patrick Christenson. He was born in 1991 and when brought to his mother, she immediately noticed one striking similarity to her first son, Kevin, who had died twelve years before, at the age of two, from cancer. Patrick had a slanted birthmark that looked like a small cut on the right side of his neck; this was the exact location where Kevin had had an operation to take out a tumor for a biopsy.

Patrick also had three unusual birthmarks that corresponded with those of Kevin's.

Then even more similarities that are unexplainable began appearing.

Kevin had limped when he was one and a half years old; Patrick started doing the same when he started walking.

When Patrick turned four and a half years old, he started talking about wanting to go back to his 'previous home'. The thing was: he'd never had a previous home — he'd lived all his life in their current home.

But his mum had indeed lived elsewhere. After Kevin's death, his mother had re-married and moved out. Despite the fact that Patrick had never seen the home Kevin had been born in, he could correctly identify it as being orange and brown.

Next, Patrick would point to the slanted birthmark and state that it was the result of surgery, though Patrick himself had not had any surgeries performed on him. It was apparent that he was referring to the surgery done on Kevin, one he wasn't even aware of.

Finally, on one occasion, Patrick saw a photograph of his brother Kevin and identified it as himself although the photograph was rarely displayed in the home.[147]

These cases seem to suggest the possibility of *reincarnation*, the idea that after death our soul takes physical form again in another body. In Chapter Seven, page 127, I mention streams of consciousness that exist independently of physical bodies. Reincarnation therefore can be taken as transference of a stream of consciousness from one body to another.

Both these cases were extensively investigated by Ian Stevenson, a Canadian-born US psychiatrist. Over the course of thirty years, Stevenson would end up collecting thousands of cases of reincarnation from around the world. His findings were published in some of the top journals in the world, including the *American Journal of Psychiatry* and *Journal of the American Medical Association*.[148]

In these cases, the children involved were often able to provide sufficient information to determine where they had lived in their previous life. Families from that previous life could be found for interviews. The child, when introduced to that family from a past life, was often able to identify accurately the members present there by their names. The children were also able to describe accurately details of events of the past known only to family members.

All this leaves us with only one logical possibility: these children had indeed been born, in a past life, to those families.

In many of these cases, the child rapidly lost these memories after six years of age, and would no longer talk about their past life after that.

As Patrick's case showed, some of the most convincing cases of reincarnation Stevenson collected involved birthmarks. For example, one boy had two birthmarks — one at the front, and another at the back, of the head — that corresponded directly to the gunshot wound that he had inflicted on himself when he committed suicide in a previous life.[149]

The most exhaustive study done on reincarnation was published in India in 2015. Since the late 1970s, a total of over 20,000 case studies on reincarnation have been compiled by more than 300 academics and scholars from over 26 countries. This document contains over 4,000 pages![150]

It is not just in research like this where proof of reincarnation has been found. There are detailed case studies from therapists working with their clients. Of course, many of these are hard to verify, but there are some that seem to show that past-life memories are not just a figment of the imagination.

Past-Life Sessions Conducted by Therapists Have Found Objective Details That Cannot be known through any Other Means

Dr. Stanislav Grof, a Czech psychiatrist, in his book *When the Impossible Happens* goes into the past-life story of Karl, a client of his.

In an experience induced through *breath work* — the conscious control of breathing to influence one's mental, emotional and physical state — Karl had visions of a fortress situated on a rock by the ocean. He also saw images of Spanish soldiers in the midst of a battle, though the scenery reminded him of Scotland or Ireland. In the vision, he saw himself as a priest with a seal ring, which was carved with some initials, on his hand.

He started to draw tentatively all the scenes he was seeing. A talented artist, he produced a number of detailed drawings, including one that depicted him being killed by a British soldier and being thrown over the fortress to lie dying on the shore. In another, he was able to draw the seal ring with the initials of the name of the priest.

On an impulse, he took a holiday in Ireland and found on his return that he had taken eleven photographs of the same location. This was surprising for two reasons: he couldn't remember having taken those photos, and the view itself was not particularly fascinating. He sought out a map, reconstructed the area he had taken so many pictures of, and discovered that all the pictures were pointing towards a ruin of an old fortress called Dun an Oir, even though the fortress could barely be seen in the photos.

When he did further research on the history of Dun an Oir, he discovered that in 1580, a group of Spanish soldiers had landed in the nearby harbor to assist the Irish in the Desmond Rebellion. Together with the Irish soldiers, numbering around 600 in total, they barricaded themselves in the fort at Dun an Oir.

Eventually they were surrounded by English soldiers led by a Lord Grey. A mediator came to negotiate with the Spaniards and promised that they would not be killed if they opened the gate and surrendered. But the English did not keep their word. Once the English soldiers were inside, all the Spaniards were cut down and thrown over the fortress onto the beach below.

As Karl probed further, he discovered a special document from the battle. The document provided evidence of a priest accompanying the Spaniards who was slaughtered together with the soldiers; the name of this priest had the same initials he had seen, encased on the seal ring, in his vision![151]

More important than these stories are the therapeutic benefits of reliving past-life memories. Many of the therapists' patients who had these past-life memories were able to connect many of their current emotional and physical symptoms to circumstances in that past-life. When these connections fully emerged into their consciousness, it often brought insights into and understanding of previously puzzling aspects of their current life. Difficult emotional and physical symptoms were sometimes totally resolved or partially alleviated.

Here's a case from a client of mine showing how past-life traumas can affect the current life.

Many Behavioral Patterns Can Be Traced to What Happened in Our Past Lives

Fanny was brought in by her husband, Leon. Still only in her 30s, she had been diagnosed with severe rheumatoid arthritis, and, with all the pains in her joints, could no longer walk properly. We had one session. Fanny recovered within a week; when she came back for a second session, she was able to walk on her own.

Trust had been established, and Fanny and Leon started showing a great deal of interest in my work. In that second session, I began reading their morphogenetic fields and found a past-life trauma in Fanny that was continuing to create stress in her body. When Fanny heard that, she got very excited and wanted me to tell her exactly what I had found.

I related to Fanny what her morphogenetic field was indicating: Fanny and her mother had been lovers in a previous life. Fanny had been the woman; her mother had been the man. In that past life, her lover had physically abused Fanny; this eventually led to her suicide in her 20s.

At this point, Leon started showing keen interest. The pattern was playing out in Fanny's current life as well: Fanny's mother had been physically abusing her from a young age. When Fanny was in her 20s, she had thoughts of suicide and had slashed her wrists.

Further probing showed that the entire family had past karmic ties to each other (which isn't surprising). Leon's father, for example, had been his son in a previous life, and Leon had been abusive towards his son. Roles had reversed in the current life, but the pattern of abuse was still there: Leon's father was now abusive towards Leon.

What finally convinced Leon was when I revealed that he had been Muslim in his last life. Thrilled, he related that throughout his life he had felt a yearning to learn more about Islam although he had been born a Catholic. For example, he felt a strong compulsion to bow whenever he heard the sound of the *muezzin* (the person appointed at a mosque to recite the call to prayer).

Controversy over Reincarnation Occurs Because Some Religions Do Not Believe That Souls Can Come Back Again

The topic of reincarnation results in huge disagreement; different religions have completely different beliefs. The *Vedas*, the four collections forming the earliest body of Indian/Hindu scripture, describe it extensively; it's an article of faith for Hindus. Other major religions that have accepted reincarnation as a doctrine include Buddhism, Jainism and Sikhism. The major religions that do not accept reincarnation comprise Christianity, Islam and Judaism (the *monotheistic* or one-God religions).

However, recent discoveries, including the Gnostic gospels of Nag Hammadi found in Egypt in 1945, and the Gospel of the Nazarenes, suggest that reincarnation may have been part of the original Bible but edited out during the Second Council of Constantinople in 553 AD, when decisions were made as to which gospels were to be considered as *canon* (the list of books officially sanctioned by the church) and which were to be considered heretical.[152] The decision was politically motivated, as reincarnation provides another chance — or several chances — for salvation. It would be difficult to sell the idea of people needing the Church with reincarnation around.

For the sake of scientific balance, we must also consider the possibility that past-life recall is merely the case of a person vibrating in resonance with another soul/consciousness living in another era, and obtaining these 'memories' through the morphogenetic field they both share. In this case, it may be true that we have only one life after all.

Regardless, in this book, for the sake of simplicity, I am going to use the labels 'reincarnation' and 'past life' for the above-mentioned phenomenon.

The most important point to note here is that a person in the current life can identify with someone else living at another time in another location, and that there is resultant transference of traumas to the current life.

So if past-life traumas set the tone for current-life traumas, like the stories of Karl, Fanny and Leon strongly indicate, what does that mean for us?

That would indicate that past-life traumas could be earlier memories on the COEX chains (Chapter Six, page 101), implying that unless we could resolve these past-life traumas, merely addressing current-life traumas would be insufficient for full healing. In fact, another story from the clinical experience of Dr. Stanislav Grof will illustrate how past lives could be shaping our birth and current-life traumas.

Past-Life Traumas Tend to Form the Earliest Memories in Our COEX Chains; it is Therefore Critical We Resolve Them for Full Healing to Take Place

Dr. Grof was conducting a group breath work session. One of the attendees was a man named Nobert who had chronic pain in his left shoulder and across his pectoral muscles. Despite many medical examinations, no causes could be found for the pain. Painkillers brought only temporary relief.

The session that Nobert participated in lasted three hours; in this time, Norbert experienced extreme pains in the chest and shoulder areas. After bouts of struggling, screaming, choking and coughing, he finally calmed down. With a start, he realized that the persistent tension across his shoulders and chest had lifted; he felt completely free of pain. The release turned out to be permanent; 20 years later, when Dr. Grof had a follow up with him, Nobert was still pain-free.

10 – Past Lives: You have lived before

Norbert's symptoms of pain in the shoulders and chest seemed to be linked to three main experiences, all involving the risk of death.

The first event he reported experiencing during the breath work session was a childhood incident in which he almost lost his life. As a seven-year old child, he had been digging a tunnel on the beach with friends. When they finished, Nobert crawled into the tunnel but it suddenly collapsed, with the sand landing hard on his shoulders and burying him. He would have choked to death if not for a speedy rescue by some nearby adults.

As Norbert's breath work deepened, the next experience he reported was during his birth when, during a difficult delivery, his shoulders jammed on the pubic bone of his mother. As a result, he experienced choking and a crippling pain in his shoulders.

Finally, in the third experience, the deepest of the session, he saw himself in a battlefield in England with soldiers surrounding him. The next thing he knew, he felt a lance piercing his shoulders. He fell off his horse and got trodden on by his panicking horse. His chest was crushed, and he eventually choked and drowned on his own blood.

Reliving this past-life experience with all its pain and distress allowed his formerly repressed emotions to be released, and brought forth deep calm and peace at the end of the session.[153]

Nobert's emotional and physical symptoms clearly show the effects of the underlying COEX chain. The COEX chain is a multilayer constellation of traumatic memories that usually begins with the current life but which can go back to ancestral-trauma memories and past-life-trauma memories. All these memories are associated with the same sensations, feelings and thoughts, all revolving around a Decision of Defeat (Chapter Five, page 87).

Summary

The stories of children below six years old who report on a past life, ie a life before their current one, is usually dismissed as fantasy by adults who hear about it.

Nevertheless, there are researchers who have done serious studies on the matter and found a great deal of evidence that the idea of reincarnation – consciousness moving from one physical body in one life to another body in another life – is valid.

If reincarnation exists, any unresolved traumas from previous lives can flow into our current life in the form of puzzling emotional and physical symptoms. When these past-life traumas are resolved, these emotional and physical symptoms often become partially or completely alleviated. The reason that uncovering past-life traumas tends to be so therapeutic is because past-life traumas are some of the earliest memories on the COEX chain, making them some of the most impactful.

Unfortunately, past lives and past-life trauma memories are still not accepted by mainstream psychiatry and psychology. Only traumas relating to our childhood and later life are accepted. Any memories from birth, ancestral and past lives are not treated as what they really are, but as possible associations with dream material or due wholly to imagination. As a result, certain therapeutic benefits are missed out.

Past-life traumas and their association with disease may seem the most controversial idea that I'm proposing in my model, since once we cross over to this realm, we have moved beyond the body and the mind into the spiritual world of death and rebirth. But I'm actually going to go one step further, into the world of spirits and earthbound entities.

ELEVEN — Spirits: Death is Not the End

Shamans View the Cause of Mental Illness as Disturbances by Spirits

Alex, an 18-year-old American, had suffered from psychotic episodes since he was 14. He had hallucinations, suicidal tendencies and severe bouts of depression. No amount of drugs or external interventions such as counselling helped. His parents were at their wit's end.

Then, through a chance encounter, Alex's family met Dr. Malidoma Patrice Somé, a shaman from Africa. Dr. Somé brought Alex back to his African village, which follows the Dagara traditions of West Africa. Eight months after being brought to Africa, Alex returned to normal. Feeling more comfortable being in Africa, he stayed on for another four years, even assisting other healers in nearby villages. Eventually he did go back to the US, and graduated from Harvard in psychology.

The reason Dr. Somé was able to help Alex, when all conventional channels had failed, was because African traditional healing systems had very different beliefs about mental illness from conventional Western ones.

Dr. Somé believes that mental illness is actually a sign of a healer waiting to be born. People with mental illnesses are super sensitive to the multi-dimensional nature of the universe, and are open to the influences of spirits from other realms. When spirits try to merge with these sensitive people, to gain an avenue for healing, symptoms such as depression, panic attacks, psychosis and hallucinations can result.

If handled correctly, through integrating these two energies (human and spirit), the disabling part of the symptoms can be eliminated or reduced, and the person becomes a healer in her own right. If handled improperly, through the administration of psychiatric drugs and institutionalization, the spirits end up tormenting the person whom they are 'supposed to inhabit', causing even more serious ailments.[154]

Dr. Somé's shamanic views may be considered superstition by many, yet Alex's results speak for themselves. Shamanism was actually the first group of therapies known to humans, but it became eclipsed by modern psychiatry.

Shamanism was Eclipsed by Psychiatry Because of the Division between Religion and Science

Before the pre-Christian era, mental illnesses were attributed to possession by evil spirits. Pre-modern cultures independently developed very similar techniques to address effectively these problems; these traditions are collectively known as shamanism. Shamans act as the intermediaries between the visible and invisible world, conducting rituals to free those afflicted.

During the scientific revolution in the 18th century (see Chapter One, page 32), conflicts arose between religious leaders and scientists. In one of the most famous examples in history, Galileo had to recant his statement, because of pressure from the Catholic Church, that our Earth went around the Sun and not vice-versa.

At that point in time, people still believed that the Sun went round the Earth. Galileo proposed an alternative model, based on scientific observations, that it was in fact the Earth that went around the sun. His statement was treated as heretical because it was believed that since humans were favored by God, all objects in Space must revolve around Earth.

A consequence of this split was that there was an uneasy compromise: anything of a spiritual nature would be handled by the religious authorities of the day while science would devote itself to physical causes.

This was the historical backdrop when psychiatry as a field was established at the dawn of the 19th century. In a bid to remove all vestiges of supernatural causes (that would have inevitably created a conflict with the Church), the focus was turned towards biological causes for mental illnesses.

Earlier practices had included bloodletting (to balance the humors in the body), insulin shock and electroshock therapy, but over time, using medication to alleviate symptoms became popular. Medication continues to be the therapy of choice in the modern world. Yet chemicals were never held out to be a cure, merely a way to make the person feel less bad.[155]

In fact, I believe that the reason *electroconvulsive therapy* — the current replacement for *electroshock therapy* — is held out as the best treatment for severely depressed patients is because the electric shock administered expels the spirit that is attached to the person.

In the late 1800s and early 1900s, a Swedish-American psychiatrist known as Dr. Carl A. Wickland wrote a book called *30 Years among the Dead* in which he described a similar protocol. He would administer a mild electric current that was too weak to cause harm to his patient but strong enough to evict the spirit from the person.[156]

The main difference between psychiatry and shamanism is that the former's philosophy has no room for supernatural causes while in the latter's philosophy, an invisible world known as the spirit world with its own inhabitants is assumed as a matter of course. So who is right: do spirits exist or are they merely figments of an overactive imagination?

Do Spirits Exist?

A survey has shown that 45-50 percent of people do believe in the existence of spirits; an even greater percentage are certain of life after death.[157] Nearly one in five people in the US have seen spirits, with almost 30 percent feeling they have been in touch with people who have passed on.[158]

So, even though sightings of or communication with spirits are so common among the general population, why do scientists remain so skeptical about their existence?

Many scientists subscribe to the view of David Hume, a Scottish philosopher who lived during the 18th century. Hume argued that we should accept something as real only if it were something our senses could pick up.

Of course, this view would seem ridiculous today. Place two magnets with their North poles facing each other; bring them close enough and they will repel each other. So we can't see magnetism, but we know it exists. We cannot sense mobile phone signals, but that does not make these frequencies any less real.

Hume asked which was more probable — for witnesses to lie about what they had seen, or for universal laws of nature to be infringed.[159] But what are universal laws of nature? As we see later when we talk about the process of death, the whole idea of spirits actually follows universal laws and is not a violation of nature.

The argument usually presented by scientists, that spirits do not exist because there is no 'scientific proof' of their existence, is also untrue.

Gary E. Schwartz, Ph.D., has done research on the existence of spirits.[160] For example, in one test using equipment to detect the number of photons in a dark chamber, he spoke to spirits and requested them to go into a dark chamber. The number of photons in the chamber was measured before the test, during the test and after the test.

When the pre-test, peri-test and post-test results were compared, it was seen that a dramatic increase in the number of photons had taken place while the spirits were inside the dark chamber.[161]

The question then becomes whether scientists will accept these findings as sufficient evidence for the presence of spirits. Arguably, scientific research in this area is still scant. However, this is also a matter of belief: since scientists have already written off the existence of spirits, no resources will be dedicated to studying the phenomenon. When someone does not want to believe in something, it's hard to persuade him otherwise, even with facts, as mentioned in Chapter One, page 34.

Even the prominent psychologist Carl Jung expressed his belief in spirits in a letter to a friend:

"I once discussed the proof of identity for a long time with a friend of William James, Professor Hyslop, in New York. He admitted that all things considered, all these metaphysic phenomena could be explained better by the hypothesis of spirits than by the qualities and peculiarities of the unconscious. And here, on the basis of my own experience, I am bound to concede he is right. In each individual case I must of necessity be skeptical, but in the long run I have to admit that the spirit hypothesis yields better results in practice than any other."[162]

Spirits are Recognized in All Cultures

Many cultures have independently created rituals to appease the souls of those who have died. For example, in Mesopotamia, burial rites involving offerings of food and drinks were common, as it was believed that a dead person could become a terrifying spirit, bringing disease, suffering and even death to the living if these offerings were neglected.

The ancient Egyptians believed in the afterlife so much that their entire civilization was predicated on the belief:

- They believed in three non-physical aspects of the body known as *ka (life-force)*, *ba* (spiritual characteristics unique to a person) and *akh (unification of ka and ba)*;

- They mummified their dead so that the soul, on returning to and reuniting with the body after it had been buried, would be able to find and recognize the body in order to live forever;

- They built elaborate tombs like the pyramids to house members of the royal family after their death.

Similarly, the ancient Hindus speak of the *atman* (the spiritual life principle of the universe), *jiva* (any entity with life-force) and *pranamayakosha* (sheath of vital energy also known as the pranic body); the Muslims of *sirr* (the innermost part of the heart), *rûh* (spirit) and *nafs* (soul); the Jews of *neshama* (soul or spirit), the *ruah* (spirit, the force or principle believed to animate living beings) and the *nefesh* (vital spirit); and the Christians of the Holy Trinity (the Father, the Son and the Holy Ghost).

The belief that spirits and entities exist is shared by all cultures and civilizations, including the tribes in Africa, the Native Americans in the American continents, and all the major religions of the East.[163] The fact that there are so many independent sources for the existence of spirits, and how they can intervene in the lives of the living, cannot therefore be a mere coincidence.

Ultimately, for the vast majority of people today, the question of the existence of spirits is not so much a matter of proof as a matter of the belief system(s) they hold.

Spirits Can Become Earthbound After Death

To understand how spirits can exist, we have to first understand the process of death.

The death process begins with what we call the 'First Death', when the physical body dies and the part of the body that is non-physical starts to separate.

Remember the Near-Death Experiences (NDEs) that I spoke about in Chapter Three (page 56)? Consciousness survives after physical death.

The non-physical body comprises several energetic bodies (see figure next page). For our current purposes, we will name just two of them: the *etheric body* and the *astral body*. The etheric body contains the template for the physical body while the astral body is what separates from the physical body during sleep to experience dream-state. In life, the astral body is connected to the physical body with a silver cord that is severed at death.

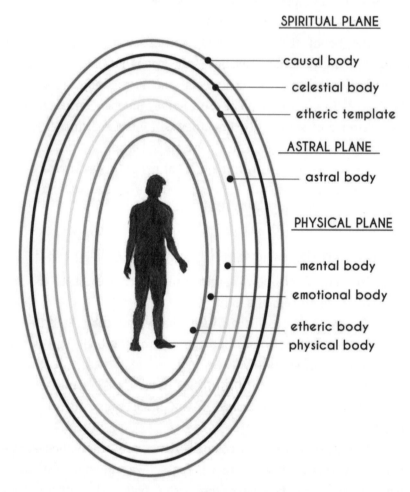

Figure 9: Energetic Bodies

The 'Second Death' happens when the etheric body dissolves, leaving behind the astral body which then moves on to the astral level. The astral level can be understood as another realm that vibrates differently from our physical world.

Between the First Death and Second Death, the etheric body continues to be aware of its surroundings and can remain active; in addition, it can subtly influence the physical world and can be 'seen' by people who are sensitive to such things.

The Second Death is supposed to occur naturally a few days after the First Death, but some spirits can stay in this intermediate state for a long time; we term these as 'earthbound spirits'.

Spirits can become earthbound for several reasons; the most common are:

- Spirits can believe they are still alive, especially if the death was sudden and unexpected;
- Spirits can still have earthly desires like an addiction for drugs, alcohol, gambling and sex;
- Spirits can believe they have done something wrong and are afraid of what will await them on the other side;
- Spirits may want revenge, especially if death was due to murder;
- Spirits may have left behind family members for whom they still feel a great attachment to.[164]

Regardless of the reason, once spirits become earthbound, they require sustenance — just as humans do from food. But unlike humans, these etheric bodies feed on energy. Someone with a similar emotional tone such as depression, anger or fear would attract these entities and cause these entities to become attached to them. This is simply the Law Of Attraction (LOA), mentioned in Chapter Seven (page 122) at work: like draws like to it.

Over time, as these spirits draw vital energy from their host, they become responsible for causing all kinds of chronic illnesses.

Children are often the first ones affected since they tend to be the most sensitive. I have discovered that the autistic children I have worked with often have at least one spirit attachment in their morphogenetic field.

Also, if a death involved disturbing circumstances like murder, suicide or abuse, earthbound spirits can remain at the place of their death, and this can have very negative effects on the people living in that place, eg a house. This is known as a haunting. For example, a person living in a house where a suicide had taken place can eventually become afflicted with severe depression and kill herself, perpetuating the cycle.[165]

What other problems do spirits cause for their hosts?

Spirits Cause All Kinds of Physical and Mental Symptoms

Whilst doing hypnotherapy, Belgium psychologist Roger Vanderdonck noticed a curious phenomenon. There was a group of 'difficult cases', people who found it difficult to enter the hypnotic state. Exploring further, he found one or more spirits attached to them.

Over the course of two years, he came across 1,131 such people; 921 had attached entities. He documented the symptoms caused by these spirits: 84 percent exhibited fatigue, 77 percent had depression, 63 percent had headaches and migraines, 60 percent suffered from neck pain or stiffness, and 23 percent had suicidal thoughts. Other symptoms he saw included digestive disorders, pain, and hearing and vision problems.[166]

How do spirit attachments create these physical and mental symptoms? Spirit attachments can attach to a person's morphogenetic or auric field. As mentioned before (Chapter 7, page 128), the morphogenetic field is critical to establishing order within the body, since it regulates many epigenetic functions and ensures that the proteins and enzymes necessary for the smooth running of the body get made.

Until they are released, these unwanted energy parasites bring their unresolved traumatic memories to bear on their host. In other words, besides dealing with your own traumatic memories, you now have another person's traumatic memories to work through. Some people have more than one spirit attachment so you can imagine the amount of stress this is likely to place on the body. This stress can manifest as nightmares, phobias and obsessive thoughts.

Shamans believe that ALL disease is caused by spirit attachments. I've come to exactly the same conclusion, based on my own work with my clients.

These Troubled Spirits are Often Ancestral Spirits Who Were Trying to Heal Their Own Issues

Most often, the spirit that attaches to a person is an ancestor or other family member, typically a grandparent, from an earlier generation. Dr. Shakuntala Modi, M.D., wrote a book called *Remarkable Healings* where she discovered that almost 92 percent of her clients had earthbound spirits; of these, 50 percent were spirits of relatives, primarily parents, grandparents, siblings, children and spouses.[167]

The motivation to attach was usually benign — concern over a family member, the belief that they could help a family member by staying with them — and the spirits had not realized that they would harm the family member in the process. Once an entity enters a person, it can't leave unless removed by people who know how to do so, ie shamans.

I wish to clarify that the ancestral spirits we are discussing here are different from the guardian angels that some sensitive people feel around them. The main difference is that our guardian angels had moved successfully into the spirit world then come back to assist us. (They may be ancestors.) Guardian angels are therefore unequivocally beneficial. The ancestors that I found who cause problems for their descendants are spirits that have not gone into the spiritual world and are still in the 'grey area' between our physical world and the spiritual world.

Spirits that are attached can occasionally move down the generations. For instance, an entity attached to a mother who has a child can transfer to the child. This is especially true for aborted or miscarried babies. Secondly, in the case of a curse, cast by a practitioner of black magic or the dark arts, that involves sending a dark entity into the family, the dark entity can continue to move down the generations until it is cast off.[168]

Dr. Somé believed that an ancestral spirit which attached itself to a body of a living descendant did so to heal some aspect of its life that it had been unable to set right whilst in its own physical body. In a way, a descendant's body becomes a vessel through which a spirit can complete its mission on Earth so as to move on to the spirit world.[169]

It is Not Necessary for Spirits to Attach to You for Illness to Strike; it is enough that Spirits were attached to your Ancestors

We established in Chapter Nine (page 151) that the (unconscious) practice of invisible loyalty can cause traumas borne by an ancestor to affect the descendants. Another way for invisible loyalty to affect a descendant is if her ancestors had spirits attached to them.

I have often encountered cases like these.

For example, I've had cases in which a client, sensing something wrong, had tried to heal herself by seeking out a shaman to do a 'spirit extraction' (ie, an exorcism in which a shaman removes the spirit attached to an aura), or a client had gone to see a medium but found no spirits in her immediate energy field.

It turned out that these attempts did not complete the healing: the person also needed to deal with the spirits that had been attached to her ancestors, even though the spirits were not attached to her, and even when her ancestors were no longer alive. (We had mentioned in Chapter 9, page 160, that ancestral traumas affect morphogenetic fields, which are not bound by space or time).

The mechanism of invisible loyalty was at play here. As long as the spirits remain attached to their ancestors, the ancestors continued to suffer, and their descendants would suffer alongside them.

There is also a common phenomenon called 'nesting' found in this kind of situations. Each generation can progressively get more and more affected through this nesting phenomenon. Let's take a look at a hypothetical case to illustrate this.

11 - Spirits: Death is Not the End

Chanel has lost a child from miscarriage. She grieves so much over the loss that she unconsciously sends a signal to the miscarried child to stay on with her even though it is supposed to move on to the spirit world. It works; Chanel now has a spirit attachment — her own miscarried child.

Over time, Chanel finds that her grief never really lets up; the spirit of the miscarried child keeps triggering that emotion in her. Eventually, Chanel has other children, but this attachment continues to live on in her field.

Over time, the attachment distorts her morphogenetic field. Chanel gets sicker and sicker; it becomes more and more difficult for her body to maintain homeostasis. She eventually dies. Because Chanel had held on to her grief while alive, it becomes much harder for her, in turn, to move on to the spirit world. Her children similarly display much grief on her death; this triggers her own unresolved grief, and her spirit chooses to stay on instead of moving on.

Say Chanel's spirit decides to attach itself to one of her children, Pauline. Pauline now has a spirit attachment from Chanel, who herself had a spirit attachment from her miscarried child.

When Pauline dies, she herself is likely to become a spirit attachment (again due to unresolved grief), so now we have the spirit of a miscarried child attached to the spirit of Chanel which is attached to the spirit of Pauline which now gets attached to someone else in the family. This is 'nesting' , the phenomenon of spirits within spirits within spirits.[170]

The best analogy for this is probably Russian dolls: open a Russian doll and you will find another smaller Russian doll within; open this smaller Russian doll and you will find yet another, etc.

So how do you know whether you have a spirit attachment or are being affected by one via your ancestral line?

Disturbances by Spirits are often Invisible and Unknown

Vanderdonck (page 186) found that of his many clients only five percent had had direct experiences of spirits that predisposed them to believe that there was a spirit presence with them.[171] For the vast majority, the spirits were a hidden influence in their life; the knowledge that they were 'possessed' would probably have been shocking to them.

Vanderdonck's way of detecting the presence of a spirit is known as the *swing-posture test*. A client would stand upright and relax. She would first be told that someone would be ready to catch her when she fell, then asked to fall in whichever direction felt most natural to her. Dropping to the right or forward was a sign for Vanderdonck of the presence of entities in her. Another test he used was feeling for temperature differences between a client's left and right sides of the neck. The left side of the neck was often colder than the right side if an entity was present.[172]

I have found that people who are affected by spirits can have unusual experiences to recount: electrostatic experiences, where electrical appliances malfunction in their presence (this is because spirits are of the electromagnetic spectrum), repeated traumatic dreams, or *sleep paralysis.*

In fact, let's look at an extreme case study where entities attached to a person could cause sleep paralysis eventually leading to death!

Sudden Unexplained Nocturnal Death Syndrome Linked to Sleep Paralysis and Entities

On a Sunday night in March 1990, Sitthi Sataisong, a 27-year-old Thai worker in Singapore, began struggling to breathe. Despite his roommate's valiant efforts to revive him, Sitthi was declared dead before dawn. At 27, Sitthi was young and healthy and had no history of heart problems. Baffled doctors had no idea what caused his sudden demise.

If Sitthi had been the only such victim of this unexpected manner of death, the situation would probably have been chalked up as a random 'act of God'. But he wasn't: 221 otherwise healthy Thai men in Singapore died suddenly of unexplained causes between 1997 and 2004. [173] A medical term has even been coined for this phenomenon: Sudden Unexplained Nocturnal Death Syndrome (SUNDS).

Singapore is not the only place where SUNDS has been seen. Researchers in the US discovered a similar phenomenon plaguing immigrants from the hill country of Laos. These immigrants, known as the Hmong, were hired as guerrillas by the Central Intelligence Agency (CIA) — the civilian foreign intelligence service of the US Government, tasked with gathering, processing and analyzing national security information from around the world — to fight the communist threat facing Laos from the late 1950s to 1975.

When they lost the war to the communists in 1975, the Hmong fled to refugee camps in Thailand to escape retaliation. More than 100,000 members of this group would eventually immigrate to the US.

In the United States, from 1977 onwards, the Hmong began to die from SUNDS. Almost all of the victims were male, in seemingly good health, and died suddenly in their sleep without any prior warning and without any known causes. Even now, after four decades of studies, SUNDS remains a mystery; no cause has been found for it.

Researchers did however notice a strange occurrence, reported by a significant percentage of the Hmong immigrants, in numbers far more than would be expected in the general population.

These Hmong reported that they often woke up during the night with an extreme sense of panic or fear, with partial or complete paralysis of their body, with a feeling of pressure on their chest, and seeing or feeling a 'presence' in the room.

In medical literature, these symptoms are indistinguishable from *sleep paralysis*. Sleep paralysis has been explained away by western medical models as a sleep disorder, with the 'presence' sensed being merely a visual hallucination. But because of the very real feeling of an entity during sleep paralysis, there is a strong belief in many parts of the world that it is spirits that are responsible for this paralysis during sleep.

In general, up to one-third of people experience sleep paralysis at least once in their life. But among the Hmong, this figure rose to an astonishing 50-60 percent after they immigrated to the US.

In the Hmong tradition, sleep paralysis is known as *tsog tsuam* (pronounced 'cho chua') and the entity that causes it *dab tsog* (pronounced 'da cho').

Interviews with the Hmong have revealed that *tsog tsuam* may provide the answer to the SUNDS mystery.

The Hmong practice animalism. This practice emphasizes the importance of offerings and rituals to be performed by the head of the household, in a bid to appease ancestors in the spirit world who then protect the family against harm by entities such as the *dab tsog*.

If these traditional rituals are ignored or broken, the *dab tsog* can cause harm by sitting on sleepers and suffocating them.

In the old tradition, when someone started feeling suffocated in his sleep, shamans were quickly summoned to help make right the situation and prevent the attacks from escalating. If this was not done, the *dab tsog* could eventually cause so much damage to the person that he would die in his sleep.

The upheavals from the civil war in Laos led to the migration of the Hmong to foreign places, and the consequent discontinuation of many of these traditional rituals. The Hmong who knew about these traditions said that SUNDS does not happen in Laos because shamans would be engaged to intervene before death could occur. In the US, however, the traditional system was no longer in place and the *dab tsog* had begun claiming victims.

Eventually, many of the Hmong, not used to an urban lifestyle, resettled into rural areas and gradually reverted to their traditional lifestyle with its ancestral rituals. This correlated with a decline in SUNDS from 1981 onwards.

In the Hmong tradition, invisible entities like the *dab tsog* are real; these entities are kept at bay when ancestral spirits are kept satisfied with rituals and ceremonies. When these ancestors are ignored, the *dab tsog* start attacking the males of the families as it is believed that the heads of the households are responsible for performing these rituals.

Materialists — people who don't believe in spirits and anything non-material — argue that genetic reasons or toxicity alone can provide a reasonable explanation for phenomenon such as SUNDS, but our 'entity theory' fits the evidence to a much greater degree than any of the scientific explanations proposed.[174]

The Hmong SUNDS story highlights a critical point: even if the allopathic medical model cannot accept the idea that sleep paralysis is caused by entities and can lead to severe harm or even death, these incidents continue to occur while mainstream researchers struggle to understand them because they are not willing to entertain the idea that the cause could be invisible, supernatural entities. A genuine scientific mindset should consider all the evidence instead of assuming that spirits can't possibly exist because they cannot normally be seen.

Similarly, if spirits are indeed responsible for causing all our illnesses and diseases, as the shamans claim, [175] then the right, scientific approach should be to explore this hypothesis instead of dismissing it without consideration.

Summary

In the view of psychiatrists and psychologists, mental illnesses have purely biological causes, eg serotonin deficiency or genetic inheritance. (Medical doctors have a similar view: physical illnesses have a biological basis.) Shamans see the situation very differently. They see all illness as a sign of disturbances by spirits.

There are two main kinds of disturbances: spirits can either haunt a place or can attach themselves to a person's morphogenetic field or aura, similar to a *parasite-host* relationship. In the latter case, the host takes on all the trauma memories of these spirit attachments. The resulting distortions in their morphogenetic field gradually deplete the host of her energy, creating symptoms such as digestive issues, fatigue and depression.

There are also trans-generational effects: even if you have no spirits attached to you, you can still be affected by them if any of your ancestors had any attached to them. In fact, many spirit attachments are ancestors who became earthbound, ie they didn't move on to the spiritual world, because of unresolved issues which they hoped to complete through their descendants.

This doesn't mean that these ancestral spirits deliberately set out to harm their descendants; more likely than not they were simply ignorant of their damaging effect on the person they got attached to.

So we have come full circle. Trauma memories create stress in the body via epigenetics mechanisms; these then lead to organ dysfunction (primarily in the gut, immune system, thyroid and adrenals), the precursors to inflammation and disease. These trauma memories can come from one's current life (womb, birth and childhood), one's past lives or one's ancestors' lives, or even from other people in the form of spirit attachments.

At this point, you may be wondering about bacteria and viruses, lifestyle factors (eg, lack of sleep), environmental factors (eg, toxins in our food), diet (eg, lack of nutrients) and exercise (eg, being too sedentary). We've been taught that these (not trauma memories) are the fundamental reasons we fall ill. Don't these cause disease as well? Don't these matter too?

These questions are addressed in Chapter Twelve and Chapter Thirteen.

TWELVE — Germs: Friend or Foe?

Antibiotics were Created on the Premise that Bacteria are the Cause of Disease

Alexander Fleming was deeply influenced by his stint in the army during World War I, when he served as a doctor in the Royal Army Medical Corps, Great Britain. He noticed many soldiers dying from hidden infections despite having antiseptics applied to their wounds. After the war, he dedicated himself to finding ways to cure disease; he believed the way to do that was to kill the bacteria responsible for the infections. He was a brilliant researcher, and his laboratory soon became well known.

In 1928, just before leaving on a holiday with his family, he placed several cultures of bacteria he had been working on on a bench in a corner of his laboratory. On his return, he noticed that one of the bacteria cultures had died while the rest were still thriving. Investigating the matter, he discovered that a fungus had killed the culture; he named it *penicillin*. Penicillin, created in the 1940s, would eventually become the first universal antibiotic for infectious diseases caused by bacteria.[176]

Antibiotics would change the face of medicine as it was then practiced. Mortality from infectious diseases fell drastically, and many people began to believe that antibiotics would finally mean the end of disease.

Of course, as we now know, that promise has not been fulfilled. In fact, bacteria seem to be winning the war. Bacteria have become resistant to antibiotics; even worse, we have the rise of *superbugs*, strains of bacteria — such as Methicillin-resistant Staphylococcus aureus (MRSA) — that have been showing up in hospitals throughout the world[177] and that are so resistant to antibiotics that the phrase 'the end of antibiotics' has become common.

In a bid to outdo the bacteria, we are creating even more powerful antibiotics. Unfortunately, bacteria are only one kind of *microbe* (microorganism); others, commonly implicated in disease, include viruses, fungi/yeast and mold. Since antibiotics are effective only against bacteria, we also need to find antivirals to deal with viruses, antifungals to deal with fungi, and so on.

All of the approaches to dealing with bacteria and other microbes hinge on one central premise: germs cause disease. They are therefore bad for us and must be eliminated from the body. The question is: is this central premise even true?

You are Probably Familiar with Germ Theory (Germs are Harmful), But There is Another Theory Known as Terrain Theory

Let's look at two people who were born in France in the 19th century. You have probably heard of Louis Pasteur because he became world-renowned for his *germ theory*. *Pasteurization*, a term we now associate with killing germs by heating milk to high temperatures, was derived from his name.

Pasteur believed that *germs* (microbes such as bacteria and viruses) cause disease. They cause disease by invading the body. In order to keep the body healthy, germs must be defended against. Germs do not change in shape or form but take on one distinct form throughout their life. They can survive on surfaces and travel through the air; that's how they are easily transmitted between people.

12 - Germs: Friend or Foe?

Does most of this sound familiar? It should, because germ theory is the paradigm that has been adopted by mainstream (allopathic) medicine.

The second person who was born in France in the 19th century is Pierre Bechamp. You've probably never heard of Bechamp, because his theory of disease, *terrain theory*, lost out to germ theory. There are many reasons germ theory won; not least is the view that since germs should be eliminated and antibiotics can do the job, antibiotics become a convenient 'cure-all', the one solution to all our problems. That is what we have been led to believe by allopathic medicine.

'Terrain' means 'whole being' in French; it refers to all the factors, situations and experiences that influence the whole being. In particular, 'terrain' refers to all the physical, emotional, mental and even spiritual experiences that may be stored in the body as cellular memories. Disease is not created by germs; germs are merely indirect causes. The true cause is a disturbed terrain. Bacteria are already present in the body; they may even aid the body in maintaining homeostasis, but they can mutate into virulent forms when the terrain is disturbed. Interestingly, Claude Bernard, Pasteur's teacher, came to similar conclusions as Bechamp.

If bacteria can mutate into virulent forms, germs are not the unchanging microbe Pasteur believed them to be. In fact, germs can change into different forms depending on the body environment they are exposed to. The official term for this is *pleomorphism* — *pleo* means many forms, *morph* means change. Pleomorphism became a hotly debated topic between Pasteur and Bechamp.[178] The allopathic model of today operates on Pasteur's belief — that pleomorphism does not exist.

Pleomorphism Proves the Terrain Theory

Bechamp believed in pleomorphism: bacteria could change

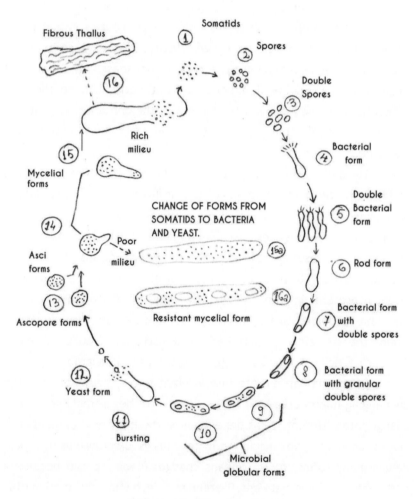

Figure 10: Pleomorphism

shape, for example, from rod-shaped to a spheroid, and change kind to become a virus or fungi. Pasteur had the opposite belief: microbes have one fixed form; bacteria, viruses and fungi are separate microorganisms.

Several discoveries support the theory of pleomorphism. French biological researcher Gaston Naessens discovered that subcellular particles in the blood, which he called *somatids* (see figure previous page), could change into sixteen different forms, including bacteria, spores and fungi, when the immune system is suppressed (refer to Figure 10).[179] German bacteriologist Guenter Enderlein discovered minute microorganisms in live blood samples that could mutate into *pathological* (disease-related) forms destructive to an organism's tissues when the organism was subjected to stress, radiation or carcinogens.[180]

Remember Rife, whom we met in Chapter Two (page 41)? The BX bacteria that he discovered seemed to be directly linked to cancer. He found that the BX bacteria are pleomorphic as well; this was later verified by Dr. Virginia Livingston and Dr. Eleanor Alexander-Jackson who wrote a paper on their findings that was presented to the New York Academy of Sciences in 1969.[181]

Why is pleomorphism such an important thing? If pleomorphism is true, it is the environment in the body that determines whether germs mutate into a form that is harmless or virulent. This is similar to the views of Rudolph Virchow, a German physician considered the Father of *Pathology* (the study of disease processes). Virchow believed that germs seek diseased tissue as their natural habitat but were not the cause of the diseased tissue, just as mosquitoes seek swamps to breed in but are not the cause of the water becoming stagnant.[182]

One example of how bacteria may not be the villains we have made them out to be can be found in the story of *Helicobacter pylori*, also commonly known as *H. pylori*. Allopathic medicine believed in the 1980s that stomach ulcers were primarily caused by a bacterial infection from H. pylori; it was also thought to be responsible for a kind of stomach cancer known as gastric carcinoma.

Thus, patients with stomach ulcers were inundated with antibiotics; as a result, H. pylori infection rates did indeed come down. In 1999, however, H. pylori was discovered to produce substances that helped kill other disease-causing bacteria like *Escherichia coli (E. coli)*. In 2001, H. pylori infections were linked with lower diarrhea rates and shown possibly to prevent another kind of stomach cancer, esophageal adenocarcinoma. This kind of cancer was rare to begin with, but it became more common after H. pylori infections fell as a result of the use of antibiotics.[183]

If bacteria are not the enemy, what is their purpose in the body?

The Purpose of Bacteria is to Help the Body to Contain Toxicity

All living things are made up of carbon, and because carbon is a finite substance, ecology has to find a way to recycle it. Microorganisms like bacteria, fungi and mold serve the function of converting carbon from one form to another, in what we call the *carbon cycle*. Specifically, bacteria and yeast act as the clean-up team while mold serves as the recycling team.[184]

What do bacteria need to clean up? They clean up toxins in the body.

12 - Germs: Friend or Foe?

We live in an increasingly toxic world. Thanks largely to the industrial revolution of the 1960s, toxins can today be found everywhere: in common foods, household products, the air and even our tap water.

There are three main categories of toxins that affect the human body:

- In terms of toxicity, the most debilitating seem to be *heavy metals* like mercury, lead and cadmium;
- Next in severity are the *xenobiotics*: man-mind substances — such as industrial compounds and chemical by-products — that mimic hormones. Xenobiotics include pesticides, solvents, and food and cosmetic additives;
- Finally, there are the *bio-toxins* released by germs such as bacteria, viruses and parasites residing in our body.

Colonies of bacteria have been found in areas of the body where there are high concentrations of mercury. It seems that the bacteria are deliberately *sequestering* (isolating) mercury.[185]

Here's a hypothesis: If the body is not able to remove toxins it has been exposed to, cells in the body start dying from exposure to these toxins. If nothing is done, the entire body gets affected and we very quickly die. The body thus allows formerly harmless bacteria to turn into a virulent form. This is a compromise solution: the bacteria help isolate the toxins from the rest of the body to prevent further damage, but the body still has to deal with the less toxic but nonetheless poisonous byproducts generated by these germs in the form of bio-toxins. So the body is literally opting for a slower death.[186]

Besides storing toxins, some of these bacteria also change into another form to help generate more inflammation in the body. What is the purpose of the inflammation? As mentioned in Chapter Two (page 49), it is to kick-start elimination by forcing the body to rest so that the body can try to eliminate these toxins more rapidly. Falling sick is the body's way of bringing itself back to balance. It's only when a condition becomes long-term that we term it 'chronic'. As the body becomes weaker and weaker, the bacteria change into more and more virulent forms to further ramp up inflammation.

Mold, on the other hand, are the decomposers in the carbon cycle. When the body becomes overwhelmed by toxicity and realizes that it can no longer cope, mold steps in to turn the body back to its most basic components — carbon — to be recycled back to earth. We call this process physical death.

So how likely is my hypothesis? Let's look at several independent findings.

Various studies have shown that cancer is a fungus.[187] When cancer tumors are biopsied, high concentrations of toxins are found. These toxins are found to be surrounded by fungus. From our earlier discussion, we can see that cancer is therefore the result of a long process in which the body tries, but fails, to counteract toxins. *Metastasis* (spreading of cancer cells) occurs because the toxins can no longer be isolated in one area of the body. Late-stage cancer is a state in which the body begins the process of breaking itself down for recycling to the dust whence we came from.

Mercury poisoning is often accompanied by the proliferation of a form of fungus commonly found in the gut, the *Candida albicans*, which binds to mercury. This explains why Candida albicans is so hard to get rid of permanently, despite repeated doses of antifungals: the body always allows the yeast to regrow as it serves the vital function of holding this heavy metal in check. Hence, killing bacteria with antibiotics or killing fungi with antifungals, without simultaneously addressing the problem of toxins in the body, is counter-productive. Once again, in our ignorance, we are fighting the body rather than assisting it.[188]

Mold has also been traced to a phenomenon known as 'sick building syndrome'. People whose immune system has been compromised often get debilitating symptoms from being around water-logged buildings which have been infested with mold (mold loves wet, dark environments). [189] Other people, with stronger constitutions, don't seem to be affected. According to our hypothesis, people who already have mold in their body tend to be more sensitive to a higher concentration of mold in their environment compared to healthier individuals who have a harmonious balance of bacteria in their body.

I hope I have established that the role of microorganisms in our body is actually to maintain the body, and, when that is no longer possible, to change form to recycle the body to its component parts to be reused again by other living beings. Germs thrive in direct proportion to the amount of toxins in the body. They are therefore just a symptom of a deeper issue of toxicity and not the cause of illness per se.

It's time to turn to some final questions you probably have about toxins.

Common Sources of Toxicity Include Dental Amalgam Fillings and Vaccinations

One of the most common sources of toxins can be found in your mouth, if you have had any dental amalgam fillings done.

Amalgam fillings are made up of 50 percent liquid mercury, one of the most toxic substances found on Earth; only plutonium, a radioactive compound, is worse.[190] It is often assumed that seafood is the culprit behind mercury absorption in humans: human industrial activity has increased the amount of mercury in the air. This eventually finds its way into lakes, rivers and the ocean, where fish and other marine life then consume it.

However, a World Health Organization (WHO) study in 1991 found that the average absorption from seafood is only 2.34 micrograms (mg) a day, whereas mercury absorption from amalgam dental fillings ranges from 3.0 to 17.0 mg per day.[191] Researchers at the Institute of Medicine at the University of Munich have found that of all the mercury found in the liver, kidneys and brain, organic mercury from seafood is quite low, at 5-8 percent, compared to inorganic mercury released from amalgam fillings, which is 95 percent, supporting the WHO study.[192]

If this really is the case, you may be wondering why dentists are putting these dental fillings in your teeth in the first place. This unfortunately is a case of history triumphing over science.

Mercury started being used in dental fillings in the 1800s because it is antimicrobial (it kills all life, including, unfortunately, us), cheap and very lasting — the shelf life of an amalgam filling in your mouth is probably the closest thing to forever you can find. No long-term study was ever performed at the time to determine the safety of putting mercury in the human body. Mercury continues to be used in dental amalgam fillings, by force of habit or by convention, by dentists.[193] Fortunately, things seem to be changing. WHO is now supporting mercury-free alternatives, with the aim of phasing out mercury not just in dental fillings but in other medical devices as well.[194]

If learning about dental amalgam fillings containing mercury has come as a surprise to you, it may well come as a shock that there is another common source of mercury in the body: vaccinations. *Thimerosal* or ethyl mercury is a preservative used in most vaccines, including Hepatitis B, DPT (Diphtheria, Pertussis and Tetanus) and flu shots.[195] In these vaccines, aluminum — an *adjuvant*, a substance that enhances the body's immune response to an antigen — is also used as an ingredient.[196] Vaccinations are another way for toxins such as mercury and aluminum to be introduced into the body.

It has been shown that mercury has a special affinity for nerves. Mercury reaches the spinal cord within the first 24 hours of administration of a vaccination jab; within another 24 hours, it reaches the brain.[197] Toxins bind to nerve endings, attack nerves and brain cells and promote inflammation.

Toxicity in the Body is the Physical Basis for All Illness

What other effects does toxicity have in the body? Metals compete with essential minerals for binding to sites on cells. As a result, toxins lead to mineral deficiencies, like zinc and magnesium deficiencies, a problem pervasive with chronically ill patients. Minerals are essential for certain biochemical detoxification reactions. For example, three hundred detoxification enzymes in the body require magnesium while zinc is essential in the operation of over ninety enzymes.[198]

In addition, xenobiotics act as hormone mimics, throwing off the delicate balance of complex interactions between the hormones. [199] Finally, toxins have been shown to influence the regulation of genes through epigenetic mechanisms. [200]

All these factors in turn enable germs to thrive in the body, as it becomes more and more poisoned. Exposure to any toxin, whether introduced from the environment or released by germs in the body, upsets homeostasis and is the underlying physical basis for all illnesses.

Recap: Stress Prevents the Body from Detoxification

We had mentioned previously (Chapter Five, page 85) that stress causes the body to no longer focus on detoxification; an organism in fight-or-flight mode is more concerned about immediate survival than on maintenance of the body through detoxification. Therefore, we can see that germs proliferate because the body is toxic; the body is toxic because stress prevents the body from detoxifying; and stress is present as a result of the traumatic memories stored in the morphogenetic field of the body. Germs are therefore not the root cause of the illness; they are merely a symptom of the illness. The real cause is the traumatic memories that are triggering the stress response.

Summary

When antibiotics were created, it was believed that diseases would finally disappear. This belief stemmed from the germ theory advocated by Louis Pasteur, that germs are the cause for disease. Another competing theory, terrain theory, was sidelined.

In terrain theory, germs are not the enemy. They are there only as a result of imbalances in the body. These imbalances are due mainly to the presence of toxicity, whether internally generated by the body or externally derived from the environment. When the body is imbalanced, the toxic environment causes germs to change form from a harmless version to one that is pathogenic to the body. The purpose is to induce inflammation to help purge toxins from the body. Germs thus serve the useful purpose of cleaning up and eventually recycling the body to carbon so that the carbon can be utilized by other living creatures.

Toxicity is ultimately the physical basis of all illnesses, so does that mean toxicity is the true cause of disease and therefore detoxification is the solution for all disease? Yes and no.

Yes, the body needs to release the toxins it has accumulated in order to ultimately be free of disease.

No, the solution is not as simple as taking detox supplements or adopting a cleaner diet.

Instead, detoxification can happen only when traumatic memories and the resulting stress response are neutralized, since it is the stress response that prevents the body from detoxifying.

Responsibility for disease has been dumped on the doorstep of not just germs but also lifestyle factors such as how much activity we get and the type of food we eat. So what is the relationship between these lifestyle factors and our health? That is the subject of the next chapter.

THIRTEEN — Lifestyle: Is Health Merely a Function of Diet and Exercise?

Biophotonic Analysis of Foods Indicates the Ideal Diet is one of Raw, Wild, Organic Vegetables and Fruits

All energy in our bodies is derived from light from the Sun. To understand this concept, let's look at our food chain. Plants draw in the Sun's rays and convert this energy into leaves and fruits, through the process of photosynthesis, with the aid of nutrients and minerals drawn from the ground. These nutrients and minerals in the ground come, in turn, from animals and plants that died in the past. As they decay, their light energy is released into the soil; this light energy is then absorbed by the plants.

These plants are then consumed by animals. Carnivores or omnivores — animals that eat other animals — therefore also ultimately derive their source of energy from the plants that their prey consumes.

Our civilization's energy is also derived from the Sun. Our electricity comes mostly from coal, oil and gas. These *fossil fuels* are the decomposed waste of animals and plants from a very ancient past. When burnt, their light energy is released and converted into useful energy.[201]

As mentioned, in the research done by Professor Popp (Chapter Seven, page 125), it is the mechanism of light, in the form of biophotons, that organizes the physical body. In the presence of stress (emotional or otherwise), the light stored by the body decreases so that over time, the body becomes sick.

Foods can therefore be evaluated based on the amount of light that they store. Professor Popp discovered that organic foods growing in the wild have twice as many biophotons as cultivated organic crops. In turn, cultivated organic crops have five times as many biophotons as commercially grown crops that use pesticides.[202]

Since the agricultural revolution of the 1970s, crops on industrial farms have typically been grown year-round with very little time for the land to lie fallow. As a result, the soil on these farms has become depleted of vital minerals. Since nutrients in the soil can essentially be regarded as stored light, the produce grown on these modern farms has lesser stored light compared to plants in the wild.

Another major problem surfacing in some of our crops is that we have been genetically modifying them to endow them with attributes that are not natural. For example, some crops have been genetically modified to produce substances that can kill their natural pests. These crops were never surveyed for their long-term impact on the health of consumers.[203]

How foods are processed can also change the amount of light stored in them. To increase the shelf life of our food, foods are routinely subjected to *irradiation* — exposure to radiation usually for the purpose of sterilization. Cooked foods, foods that have been irradiated and microwaved foods, and processed or fast foods, have been found to have almost zero biophotons.[204]

Based on the biophotonic analysis of foods, then, foods should be eaten wild as much as possible, or at least grown through organic means. Foods should also be eaten raw (not cooked) as much as possible.

Raw Foods Reduce the Enzymes needed to be Secreted by the Pancreas for Digestion

Advocates of raw-food diets espouse them not on the basis of biophotonic analysis but on their enzyme potential for the human body. This is just another perspective, another way of evaluating the kinds of foods that are good for us. To digest our foods properly, enzymes are needed. Some of these can come from the foods we eat while others have to be produced by our own body.

Food enzymes present in raw food include *proteases* for digesting protein in meat, eggs and cheese; *lipases* for digesting fats in dairy products and meats; and *amylases* for digesting carbohydrates, starches and sugars. The additional enzymes obtained from raw foods help not only with digestion but with cleansing the body by breaking down allergens and harmful environmental products.

However, cooking food beyond 40 degrees Celsius (105 degrees Fahrenheit) causes a rapid deterioration in the effectiveness of the enzymes in the food. Cooked food therefore places a greater strain on our pancreas to supply the necessary enzymes to aid in the digestive process. In fact, raw foods get digested in around one-third to half the time of cooked foods.[205]

There are Arguments for Both Vegetarianism and Meat-Eating

Besides plants we also have meat, of course. There are very different viewpoints on whether people should be having a purely vegetarian diet or a diet comprising both vegetables and meat.

Several studies seem to show that becoming a vegetarian — and even more so a *vegan* (eliminating all animal-based products such as milk, cheese, eggs, and gelatin) — is the healthier way to go. By eliminating all meats and dairy, you increase the likelihood of living a long, healthy life. Eating processed meats — those that are preserved through smoking, curing or salting, or through the addition of chemical preservatives — seems to pose the biggest risks. Processed meats often contain toxins that have been shown to increase cancer risk, especially bowel cancer.[206]

There is a counter-argument from Dr. Weston A. Price who studied primitive cultures and came to the conclusion that none of these cultures were strictly vegetarian, although they did emphasize nutrient-rich foods, whether plant- or animal-based.[207]

Therefore, there appears to be no diet that fits everyone across the board. Others, in particular a person known as William Wolcott who conceived the idea of the Metabolic Typing Diet, have made similar claims.

Metabolic Typing Diets are determined by Environmental Factors, Including Stress Experienced by Ancestors

William Wolcott, a pioneer in customized nutrition, discovered there are three kinds of metabolic types: the protein-type, the carbohydrate type and the mixed type. People who are more suitable for the protein-type diet are termed carnivores while people more suitable for a greater intake of carbohydrates are known as vegetarians.

These metabolic types are based predominantly on hereditary factors and the geographic region that a person hails from. For example, during winter in temperate climates, it was impossible for plants to grow, so meat became the only option. People who live in latitudes far from the equator tend to follow the protein-type diet because meat is the only food available to them during the harsh winter months.

Near the equator, though, plants are found year-round so food sources have generally been grains. Hence, people residing near equatorial latitudes tend to do better on the carbohydrate-type diet.[208] If you think this sound suspiciously like epigenetics — bingo! I came to a similar conclusion.

I believe that the mechanism for these different diets is indeed epigenetic in nature. The further north or south from the equator you go, the less is the light received by plants on a yearly basis. People who live in these northerly or southerly latitudes cannot possibly receive enough light from the sun merely by eating plants, and therefore their body has adapted to deriving light from eating meat instead.

As mentioned in Chapter Five (page 83), the autonomic nervous system controls metabolism, and is affected by stress. My hypothesis is that the stress that a person (and his ancestors) has received will affect his metabolism, the biochemical changes that result, and therefore the kind of diet that is suitable for him.

Based on the discussion above, we have established the general principle of a good diet: eating foods that store more light. Typically this would be raw foods, especially organic raw vegetables and fruits.

However, another element to consider is the inherent hereditary factor: the genes of an individual based on the geographical location she is born in. The influence of epigenetics means that the type of foods that are more suitable for a person would depend on the environment of her ancestors, and hence the diet of her ancestors. This presumably includes the stresses that her ancestors have experienced and how they have coped with these stresses.

All of these factors come together to cause a person to develop a particular metabolic type that then determines the proportions of meat, vegetables and carbohydrates that is most suitable for her to consume as part of her regular diet.

Ultimately, the idea is still to obtain light from the foods a person eats; it's just that for some people (especially those living away from the equator), meat is also a good source of light as their body has adjusted to metabolize it.

A third factor to consider when deciding on a suitable diet is the presence of food intolerances or allergies to certain foods.

Food Intolerances are a Sign of Digestive Problems

Melanie has been in constant pain for the past few years. She has taken painkillers to no avail. Her joints have been almost-perpetually inflamed, and she has had constant neck, shoulder and back tension. When she was tested, her food-intolerance list was so long that it was almost impossible to find something she could consume without some kind of strong autoimmune response. As a result, she suffers from constant, widespread inflammation and pain. Melanie can trace these to a childhood in which gastric and heartburn symptoms were common. Her issues with food have only worsened with age.

People with any chronic illness have a condition known as leaky gut syndrome that arises from a persistent stress response in the body (Chapter Four, pages 74 and 75: persistent stress response → elevated cortisol levels → leaky gut syndrome → chronic inflammation → chronic illness).

Foods that are not digested properly, especially gluten (a mixture of two proteins found in cereal grains, especially wheat) and casein (the main protein in milk), can enter the bloodstream through the porous lining of the gut, causing the immune system to get activated and attack these substances in the blood, causing inflammation in the body.

Besides gluten and casein, other food substances I have found that seem to cause problems for many people include:

- Broccoli, spinach and other cruciferous vegetables (which seem to suppress thyroid function);
- Hazelnuts and walnuts (these should be soaked overnight first to allow them to be digested more easily);
- Chicken and eggs (from the growth hormones injected into chickens in industrial farms);
- Nightshades (vegetables such as potatoes, and fruits such as eggplant, tomatoes and peppers) which cause inflammation in the joints if a person has severe leaky gut; and
- Seafood such as mussels, oysters, prawns and crabs.

Food intolerances should be distinguished from food allergies; the effects of food intolerances usually take a longer time to show.

For example, up to 1 percent of the world's population is allergic to peanuts. [209] Indeed, for some people, the allergic reaction from peanuts can be fatal and the effect is usually immediate. However, in the case of food intolerances, eg intolerance to the gluten from wheat, it may take up to a day before the effects start to show in the body. Because cause and effect is not so clear, people have a harder time knowing what food intolerances they have.

The first thing a person who is sick usually does is restrict her diet. Will that work? Would eliminating wheat and dairy, or other 'usual suspects', from the diet help?

Of course it would: digestion takes up a lot of energy. Therefore, reducing foods that are hard to digest would help the body to utilize the saved energy for other purposes, detoxification for example. However, as the example with Melanie shows, as a person gets sicker, more and more foods become out-of-bounds. To cut out all food is clearly impractical.

Food intolerances and allergies, just like the matter of the type of diet most suitable for an individual, seem to be merely symptoms of a bigger issue: stress affecting the gut. In fact, stress changes the 'balance of bacteria' (the number of good bacteria versus the number of bad bacteria) in the gut, which then affects digestion and absorption. Chronically ill people have low levels of Vitamins B6 and B12 in their bodies because these vitamins are made by the bacteria in the gut.[210] These B vitamins are in turn crucial for detoxification.

I can extend the argument (about eliminating unsuitable foods) to removing foods that get converted to sugar quickly (known as *high glycemic-index* foods), because of their potential to cause or worsen diabetes, but as mentioned in Chapter Four (page 75), insulin production has a lot to do with hormonal imbalance issues, again as a result of stress.

What's my point in the last four paragraphs?

The Kind of Food We Eat is a Contributor to Disease, Not the Cause of Disease

I want to make an important distinction: is something the *cause* or merely a *contributor* to disease? When it comes to diet, my belief is that it is the latter, not the former.

Stress seems to be the underlying cause of leaky gut syndrome; leaky gut syndrome is then responsible for food sensitivities and allergies. In addition, based on our discussion at the beginning of this Chapter, we receive light from our environment through foods and sunlight. Stresses deplete our light storage because the DNA needs to send out more biophotons to organize our body in response. If the total light received from our food sources and sunlight is less than the light lost from stress daily, then over time we begin to suffer from a net deficit of light. This loss of light means that the body is not able to continue to organize itself, causing disease over time.

Therefore, the foods we take do not by themselves cause disease. (Of course, we are not referring to extreme examples like starvation, a situation in which light is lost without being replaced). They either promote health (when the biophoton content in them is high), or worsen an existing health situation (when the biophoton content in them is low) as there is nothing to counteract the biophotons lost from stress. In other words, diet can increase or retard the progression of disease, but it is very unlikely to reverse it totally because it never was the cause of those disease conditions in the first place.

My experience is that even the most wholesome and appropriates diets do not, by themselves, resolve an illness when the stress process has been well underway.[211] However, it does support the body's recovery and slows down the progression of diseases. That also applies to exercise.

Exercising Help to Combat the Effects of Stress, But It's *Not* Lack of Exercise That Causes Disease

Exercises have been found to increase the production of a protein known as brain-derived neurotrophic factor (BDNF). BDNF is a growth factor that helps to build neurons in the brain and is crucial for brain health because it protects the brain against the inflammatory effects of cortisol.[212] Yes — the same cortisol involved in the stress response mentioned in Chapter Four (page 73).

You probably know where I am going with this. Is exercise and activity important? Yes, definitely. Besides increasing the BDNF protein, exercise helps stimulate the lymphatic system. This system — unlike the circulation system which has its own pump (the heart) — depends on movement and exercise to move waste materials in the lymphatic system out of the body. Therefore, exercise and activity help in detoxification.

In addition, in Chapter Five (page 86) we spoke about how a person can be stuck in the sympathetic state — the stress response state, activated when a threat is deemed to be present — because excess energy is not discharged from the body after a trauma. Exercise, if done with awareness, can help discharge the excess energy, provided the trauma memory is accessed and worked through the body.

Nevertheless, we are looking at the causes of disease, and not exercising is not a cause. Exercise merely helps protect the body against the effects of stress after the stress response has *already* been activated. In some cases, over-exercising can even aggravate the stress response.

Summary

One of the things that happens as a result of stress is a change in our metabolism. This change in our metabolic state influences the diet that is most suitable for us. At a macro-level, we are also influenced by the type of diet that our ancestors adapted to over many generations because of the environmental and geographical conditions they endured and the resulting stress effects on their metabolism. We optimize our health if we eat foods that our ancestors ate in the past; our health may suffer if we don't.

From the perspective of the light stored in food, the diet most suitable for us is the one that most increases the amount of stored light in our body. This, as a general rule, is best obtained from wild, raw, organic vegetables and fruits. However, this ideal diet has become modified by changes that occurred in our metabolic type because of epigenetic changes.

From these examples, we can see that there doesn't seem to be a one-size-fits-all diet that would suit everyone.

For food intolerances and allergies, we see a similar pattern at work. Stress weakens our digestive system and the digestive lining, causing undigested foods to enter into our bloodstream and resulting in inflammation response. In this leaky gut condition, foods that are hard to digest therefore worsen inflammation.

Exercise has been shown to reduce the effects of inflammation on the body, which is the reason why people who exercise regularly feel better in many ways. However, it's like running on an endless treadmill: the moment you stop exercising, stress creeps up again and rears its ugly head.

If exercising and eating the right foods could address the true causes of diseases, we would expect people who are health-conscious to be in good health. Unfortunately, you probably can see — from your own attempts or those of someone you know — that this is not true.

We are confused about what the true causes of our illnesses are, because we have confused cause — what creates disease (stress) — with contributors — poor diet and lack of regular exercise and activity. A good diet and regular exercise and activity can help reduce the stress response and associated inflammation, but it cannot completely resolve them.

The different methods for addressing the true causes of disease will be covered in my next book *Reversing the Disease Code*.

The metabolic typing diet highlights how our ability to digest certain foods is linked to how the environment over time has epigenetically changed the genes of our ancestors. So what is the relationship between our environment and our health? In the next chapter, we explore how an individual both is affected by the environment and *influences* the environment via her consciousness.

FOURTEEN — Environment: Do We Shape the Environment or Does the Environment Shape Us?

All Living Things Derive Order from the Sun

Alexander Chizhevsky, a Belarusian scientist, was a dashing young man of 25 when he published a book in 1922. The book, called *Physical Factors of Historical Process*, made the then-outrageous claim that our behavior can be adversely shaped by the activity of the Sun. He stated, in particular, that the Russian Revolution of 1917 was incited by *solar maximum*, a period where there is a peak in sunspot activity.

This claim didn't sit well with Joseph Stalin when he took over the reins of Russia, and Chizhevsky was banished to prison for eight years in 1942 for writing the book, amongst other 'crimes'.

Despite all the opposition he faced throughout his life, Chizhevsky painstakingly continued his research, checking records of major upheavals like wars and revolutions that had occurred over two thousand years in seventy-one countries. He found that more than 75 percent of them happened during a solar maximum. [213] Further research after his death in 1964 also found a fifty-six-year cycle for financial crises linked to the cycles of the Sun and Moon; even acts of terrorism were found to correspond to these Sun and Moon cycles. [214]

A solar cycle lasts for approximately eleven years. First there is a build-up phase, when solar activity starts to increase, and then there is a decline, when sunspots reduce in intensity. Solar activity has a direct effect on Earth's magnetic field; we'll discuss this in detail later when introducing *geopathic stress*.[215]

Solar activity has a deep impact, at the cellular level, on all living beings so it should not come as a surprise that it affects our behavior as well. Franz Halberg, a Romanian biologist who coined the term *circadian rhythm* in the 1950s, noticed that many different functions of our body — including our heart variability, pulse rate, blood pressure and body temperature — follow a cycle that is linked to the Sun.[216]

Solar maximums seem to affect our sympathetic system and activate our stress response. During solar maximum, heart attacks rise, and there is an increase in all kinds of psychiatric conditions and hospitalizations, seizures, epilepsy fits, cases of sudden infant death syndrome and suicides. In particular, the number of suicide cases and the severity of depression cases seem to follow a solar wind cycle that lasts approximately 1.3 years. It has even been linked to our size at birth: if you are born during solar maximum, you are likely to be larger.[217]

I brought up the biophotonic properties of living beings earlier (page 125); biophotons explain how solar activity can affect living organisms.

The originator of quantum theory, Erwin Schrödinger, who obtained the Nobel Prize in physics in 1933, believed that there is an underlying organization in a living organism because it is constantly in the process of exchanging information and deriving order from its environment. To Schrödinger it was sunlight that provides this information and order.

This applies not just to plants and the familiar process of photosynthesis but also to animals and humans as well. All living beings use this light drawn from the Sun to provide order for themselves.[218] In other words, human beings are not just individuals isolated from their environment. Our environment is also shaping our health and us. We know that plants grow by using sunlight and nutrients from the earth, but we probably don't realize that humans are in many aspects the same: we are in balance through our interaction with the Sun and Earth.

Besides receiving information from the Sun, we also rely on the electric and magnetic fields coming from Earth.

There is a Natural, Health-enhancing Earth Frequency of 7.83 Hz

In 1952, German physicist Winfried Otto Schumann predicted mathematically that Earth should be emitting natural, extremely low frequencies, now known as *Schumann resonances*. In 1954, Schumann and his colleague H. L. König discovered that the lowest frequency mode of the Schumann resonances occurs at a frequency of around 7.83 Hz.

This frequency, now known as the Schumann Frequency, seems to have a healing effect on people. Robert C. Beck, a US physicist, performed experiments with healers from different faiths and regions, including Native-American shamans, Christian faith healers and Hindu yogis. He found that the brain wave frequency of all the healers shifted to around 7.83 Hz while the healing was occurring.[219]

If people are taken out of the natural earth magnetic field — for example, when astronauts go into space — they soon suffer from all kinds of mental and physical symptoms. In an experiment, student volunteers were recruited to live for a month in an underground bunker built to screen out all magnetic fields. The students soon began showing signs of emotional distress and migraine headaches. Their health was restored only when they were exposed to the Schumann Frequency of 7.83 Hz again.[220]

In addition, if a person is living in a home where the frequency coming from Earth is not 7.83 Hz, health issues can manifest. The Chinese have always believed that disharmony between the individual and his home can affect health, relationships and prosperity; the study of this is known as Feng Shui. The Indians have a similar tradition known as Vaastu.

Geopathic Stress occurs When the Body becomes affected by Distorted Earth Energies

The most common reason Earth's natural frequency becomes distorted is because of tectonic fault lines or underground river streams. The term coined for this phenomenon is *geopathic* (*geo* meaning earth, *pathic* meaning causing illness) stress. A related phenomenon is *electrosmog*: man-made electromagnetic fields emitted from our electronic equipment and wireless devices. Both of these fields can distort morphogenetic fields and hence affect our health.

In particular, geopathic stress areas have been found to not only cause illnesses but also nullify any treatment a person may be undergoing. In fact, different experts in the field of geopathic stress have claimed that it contributes anywhere from 30 percent to 100 percent of all disease, including all cancers.[221] These researchers are currently being taken very seriously in Europe, especially in Germany and the UK.

The reason geopathic stress can lead to disease is that electromagnetic emissions from Earth can alter the *optical polarity* of molecules of blood. Organic molecules can come in one of two forms: the 'L form or the 'R' form, so named because they cause polarized light to rotate to the left or the right, respectively. All living things naturally have the 'L' form; for example, amino acids come in the L-arginine or L-tryptophan forms. The 'R' forms cannot be used by the body.

When molecules in the blood are exposed to geopathic stress, amino acids can switch from the natural 'L' form to the unusable 'R' form. Without a usable form of amino acids, there is a deficiency in some of the proteins needed for important cellular functions. This phenomenon is also found in cancer sufferers, hence the assertion that geopathic stress is a factor in cancer formation.[222]

So, on first sight, geopathic stress seems to be a matter of bad luck. If we are unfortunate enough to be sleeping in a room or living in a location where geopathic stress exists, too bad; it appears our only recourse is to move the bed, sleep in another bed (both still practical) or move homes (worst-case scenario).

That was what I thought too, until I met Madeline ...

Geopathic Stress and Electromagnetic-Field Stress Seem to be related to the Presence of Entities

When Madeline and her autistic son, Lionel, came to see me, the stress in her son's body seemed to be associated with geopathic stress and *electromagnetic-field stress* (stress from the electromagnetic fields emitted from very-low-frequency electrical and electronic appliances such as TVs, refrigerators and washing machines).

I gave her the standard advice that in these cases is to move the bed to avoid these fields. Madeline did what I asked her to, but the next time I saw Lionel the stress was still present when I checked his morphogenetic field. To clear the mystery, I decided to visit their home to find out for myself what was happening.

In their home, I found a geopathic stress line (which is invisible and can be detected only by *dowsing*, a kind of energy test) cutting directly under the part of the bed where Lionel's stomach normally lay when he was sleeping. I asked what they did at night before going to bed; Madeline replied that she would usually turn the fan on. I got her to switch on the fan; the moment she did a ball of energy (again invisible) appeared right in the middle of Lionel's bed, over the area his stomach would usually be when he was asleep.

Madeline then told me a story that made everything fall into place. Madeline and her husband had tried to have children for a long time but had failed, so they had finally opted for in-vitro fertilization (IVF). Three attempts were made; of these, two fetuses didn't grow to full term. Lionel was the only one to be born successfully.

14 - Environment: Do We Shape the Environment or Does the Environment Shape Us?

The two fetuses that didn't make it became earthbound; they made up the ball of energy I saw in Lionel's bed. Apparently, the two spirits were absorbing the electrical energy discharged when the fan was turned on. This strengthened their etheric bodies; it also created the electromagnetic-field stress. As I had mentioned in Chapter Eleven (page 185), spirits draw etheric energies from the environment or emotional energies from people to sustain themselves.

When I sent the spirits off to the spiritual world, the geopathic stress and the electromagnetic-field stress *disappeared as well*. This was a revelation for me. This could mean only one thing: earth energies are neutral — they become distorted only because of the presence of entities in the area. It's the consciousness of these entities that causes geopathic and electromagnetic-field stresses.

Six months later, when Madeline and Lionel came to see me again for a follow up, Madeline pronounced that Lionel had shown tremendous improvement since that clearing.

It is interesting to note that in Lionel's case, as well as in many other cases I've seen of geopathic stress lines affecting health, the geopathic stress lines tended to cut through the body's gut area, where 80 percent of the immune system is.

Let's now piece together the pieces of the puzzle:

- If indeed spirits are associated with all disease (Chapter Eleven, page 186);
- If all disease is linked to problems with the digestive system (Chapter Four, page 78); and
- If, as some geopathic stress experts believe, geopathic stress is the cause for all illness (this Chapter)

- Then all three phenomena (spirits, digestive system problems and geopathic stress) are actually one and the same, just couched in different terms.

In other words, the absence or presence of geopathic or electromagnetic stresses is *not* luck or coincidence; geopathic or electromagnetic stresses are present in a home when someone is accompanied by ancestral spirits (which, remember, are unaware that their presence is contributing to their descendant's lack of health). The presence of these spirits weakens the immune system of the person; this eventually manifests in disease.

Our Consciousness Shapes Our Environment

The example of geopathic stress above helps to explain a key aspect of how our environment affects our health. We are not just helpless victims subjected to the whims of the environment; our consciousness can shape our environment (another way of expressing this is that "Our thoughts create our reality").

It's time for a recap. The principle of resonance — another way of saying the Law of Attraction — states that our environment is nothing more than a creation of our thoughts. Of course, these thoughts are often unconscious, and they may not come from our current life. All of us are made up of strings that are vibrating (Chapter Seven, page 122). The more closely two strings are vibrating with each other, the more they resonate. Through resonance, things with a similar vibration as ours are drawn to us and become our reality.

This law is universal; it applies whether we happen to be living in a home that is haunted or a mold-infested home, and it applies when we experience an accident (recall the pattern in Anne Ancelin Schutzenberger's family, Chapter Nine, page 151).

Our Environment Provides the Triggers for Our Illnesses

Our consciousness shapes our environment, which then shapes our consciousness in how we interpret and perceive events through the decisions we make. Interpreting a traumatic event through a Decision of Defeat (Chapter Five, page 87) sets us up for similar future incidents that continue to vibrate in resonance with our disempowering decision until we make a new, more loving, more empowering decision. Each event in our life is therefore an opportunity for us to make a new choice about how we perceive the situation.

We all have the capacity to withstand stress and pressure. Depending on the degree of stress that affected our ancestors, and, through the mechanism of ancestral / trans-generational traumas, the stress we 'inherited', we are all predisposed to having a particular constitution that will determine how much stress we can withstand before our body breaks down.

Imagine a barrel. If the barrel is full of water, any additional water you pour into it would simply spill over the sides. If the barrel is empty, a lot of water can be poured into it before the same thing happens.

In this analogy, your body is the barrel and the water is the amount of stress affecting you. How full the barrel is to begin with depends on your ancestry, your past-life traumas and the number of spirits that are attached to you and your ancestors. If your barrel is very full it requires just a little amount of water (stress from current-life traumas) to tip you over the edge. (This is the case of people who have been physically ill from a very young age.) If your barrel is very empty, you are blessed with a hardy physical constitution and you can take a lot of stress in the course of your life before you succumb to illness.

The water that fills up the barrel is also known as 'triggers'. Triggers can be environmental or emotional in nature. For example, an environmental trigger could be a vaccine that leads to the onset of autism in a child when the vaccine is administered to him. It is often the final load that "breaks the camel's back". We probably also know someone who started having a chronic illness after a period of intense emotional stress in her life, for example after a divorce or the death of her husband. Triggers don't happen randomly; they occur to someone because of his consciousness, through the Law of Attraction.

There have been many arguments about nature versus nurture when it comes to disease. You now understand that both nature and nurture are involved. Nature is represented by our genetics, epigenetics and our predisposition (via our ancestry) to carry vulnerabilities for some diseases, but in order for disease to take root, we need a trigger or several triggers (nurture). These triggers affect us where we are most vulnerable as a result of our emotional characteristics (Chapter Six, page 105).

For instance, a person has an accident (an environmental factor) and suffers a whiplash. As a result, she suffers from continuous neck pain. We can see the accident as separate from her consciousness; that is just the way many people would see it. However, the person who had the accident has probably been harboring thoughts of resentment towards or annoyance with certain people; the accident is merely a manifestation of her consistent thought patterns. As she has people in her life who are a 'pain in the neck' (a nuisance), she attracts to herself the accident and the whip-lash. This then causes her to experience physical 'pain in the neck'.

To develop this further, these feelings of resentment and annoyance were set in motion by earlier incidents in birth or childhood, or even by unresolved feelings that her ancestors had experienced when they were alive.

Thus, our consciousness shapes our environment that then shapes our consciousness, in an endless cycle we call life.

Summary

Human beings derive order and receive health-affirming impulses from the environment, especially through the Sun and Earth.

Solar flare discharges or a distortion in the Earth's electromagnetic fields where one is living, working or sleeping, on the other hand, can cause serious illnesses over time. The existence of this distortion in the earth fields, known as geopathic stress, is found to be highly correlated with disease.

The conventional view is that if you experience geopathic stress where you live you need to move bed or home. My hypothesis, quite different from the conventional view, is that earth fields are by themselves neutral. It is the consciousness of the person (and possibly the consciousness of entities attached to the person) living in the area that activates the earth fields and make them either health affirming or disease causing.

If this is true, our consciousness has shaped the environment we are in. Our consciousness is the sum of all decisions made by our ancestors and us. We then attract circumstances that fit our consciousness based on the Law of Attraction. If these circumstances are traumatic, they can trigger a stress response that adds to our existing set of stresses from previous traumatic memories. If the accumulation of these stresses exceeds the 'stress capacity' of our body, the disease process is initiated.

Furthermore, these circumstances cause us to make new decisions, which then attract future similar experiences. There is a never-ending *feedback loop* of our consciousness influencing our environment that then influences our consciousness.

In this Chapter, we saw how the individual can influence the environment through her consciousness. In the next chapter, we are going to look more carefully at the relationship between human consciousness and a higher consciousness, and the huge implications that link has for our health.

FIFTEEN — Holons: Higher-Order Systems Organize Lower-Order Systems

All Living Things are influenced by Galactic Events

Geobiologists (scientists who study both geology and biology) have noticed a very curious phenomenon.

Every 26 million years, life undergoes a mass extinction; the creatures that survive this extinction seem to evolve to a higher level. (Another cycle length that has been proposed for mass extinctions is 62 million years.)

This phenomenon is known as 'punctuated equilibrium': animals don't seem to evolve slowly and gradually as advocated by *Neo-Darwinists* (believers in Darwin's theory of natural selection) but in short bursts of evolution followed by a long period of stability.

Dr. Bruce Runnegar, an Australian astrobiologist from UCLA, discovered that around 65 million years ago, at the time of the mass extinction of the dinosaurs, there was also a "chaotic change in the resonant frequencies of the Solar System" which threw the planets in our solar system out of their original orbit. It is also in that period, they believe, that the single landmass previously present on Earth (Pangaea) finished breaking apart, creating the continents we know today. [223]

If mass extinctions have been regularly happening over an extended period of time, could this mean that, just as the Sun influences the planets and all beings on it, our solar system is similarly affected by galactic events of a cyclical nature?[224] How is this relevant to our discussion?

In Chapter Eight, while discussing genes, I established that DNA is actually energetic (page 136) and expresses itself based on information that DNA is tapping from morphogenetic fields (page 141). Could the massive changes in the evolution of species be caused by a change in morphogenetic fields brought about by galactic waves that bring new information into the morphogenetic fields and help guide the expression of DNA for all living things?

If so, these galactic events, with their 'galactic-wave effect' (similar to the solar flare effect), disrupt not only our physical environment but also our body's energetic systems, leading to a transformation of our consciousness.

This appears to be the best explanation proposed to explain punctuated equilibrium and the evolution of all living beings on Earth.

Consciousness can be divided into Higher-Order Systems and Lower-Order Systems, and Higher-Order Systems Organize Lower-Order Systems

In the earlier Chapters, we focused on how causes of disease in an individual are conventionally traced to the individual's stress levels because of the common belief that the causes of disease are only personal, that it is our individual thoughts and emotions that shape our body.

However, from our discussion on ancestral / trans-generational traumas and epigenetics in Chapter Nine (entire Chapter), we see that we are also intimately affected by events that happened to our family of origin. The reason our family of origin can affect us relates to the fact that there is a consciousness that we call the 'family soul'.

Let's use the term 'individual soul' for the consciousness of an individual. By extension, our family would have a family soul, our country a country soul, and so on.

It's time to look more closely at this 'consciousness' I've been speaking about since Chapter One of this book.

All spiritual and religious traditions agree that there is a Higher Power. It has been called 'God', 'Creator', 'Source' and many other names. As the words 'God' and 'Creator' have religious connotations, I'll be using the more neutral term 'Source' to refer to this Higher Power from now on.

If all of us are made up of strings that resonate and have consciousness, then Source — which comprises everything in existence — is a combination of all the strings. Source also has to be present in the universe, our galaxy, the solar system, our Sun, Earth, humanity, our country, our race, our family and also us. It must also be present in every cell of our body.

We define a higher-order system as being made up of lower-order systems. Thus the family soul includes all the individual souls, while all the individual souls together constitute the family soul.

The higher-order system organizes the lower-order system, while issues in the lower-order system are ultimately reflected in the higher-order system. Thus, the health of each individual in the family is organized by the family soul because the family soul is the higher-order system. Any trauma memories held by any individual soul in the family would also become reflected in the family soul and can therefore affect another individual soul in the same family.

As we step up the ladder of consciousness, events that have happened or are still happening to our community, our country, humanity, Earth, the solar system and even the galaxy, can affect us because we are a part of all of these successively higher-order systems.

Hermes Trismegistus wrote this in the Emerald Tablet: "As above, so below. As within, so without."[225] What is happening 'above' — for example, in our galaxy — is reflected in the lower-order systems 'below': our solar system, Sun, Earth and us. Perhaps astrology, or the study of how stars and planets can affect individuals, has a basis after all. In addition, what is happening 'within', in our consciousness, is reflected in the 'without' of our environment (we covered this in the previous Chapter).

We appear to be living in a holographic universe (Chapter Seven, page 116). Arthur Koestler, a Hungarian-British writer, coined the term *holon*, something that is simultaneously both a whole and a part. Holons are autonomous (independent) units that are free to function as a whole in their own right yet are also part of a bigger whole and thus subjected to control by one or more higher 'authorities'.

If we do live in a holographic universe then every lower-order system is just a holographic reflection of a higher-order system. In other words, a cell in our body reflects the entire universe. What is within the cell is thus reflected without, in our universe.[226]

In nature, this self-similar nature is reflected in the phenomenon of *fractals*. Objects in nature seem to follow a similar pattern at different scales, from the very small to the very large, and can be built up by repeating a similar pattern at higher and higher scales.

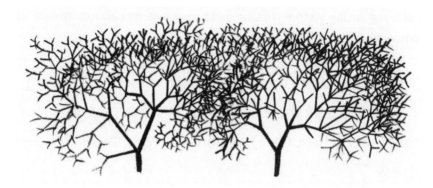

Figure 11: Trees as a Representation of Fractals

An excellent way of understanding this is to look at a tree. In a tree, the twigs or smallest branches can be regarded as the lowest-order system of the tree. These smallest branches develop off large branches that can be thought of as higher-order system of the tree. Finally, we have the main trunk of the tree from which all the large branches grow; the trunk can be seen as the highest-order system of the tree.

(We can continue this progression by looking at a tree as a lower-order system of a forest.)

Some scientists have proposed the idea that we live in a fractal universe.[227] I agree.

Let's look at one particularly important higher-order system affecting the health of every one of us on planet Earth: the Earth Soul, known as Gaia.

The idea that our Earth was a living consciousness was proposed as early as the 1970s by the English chemist James Lovelock and co-developed by the US microbiologist Lynn Margulis (and by ancient traditions millennia ago). In the Gaia hypothesis, the Earth is a self-regulating system that helps to maintain equilibrium within all forms of life on Earth.[228]

Overpopulation of Humans is Adversely Affecting the Earth, and the Earth Soul is righting the Imbalance through Creation of Traumas and Stress

According to a Norwegian legend, lemmings search for their lost Atlantic continent home by marching into the sea in an act of collective suicide.

This legend came about after noticing that every three or four years, lemmings would undergo a 'migration' that has now been established to be the result of overcrowding. The overcrowding leads to stress — lesions have been found in the brain and adrenals of these creatures — which then leads to behavior that can only be considered 'psychotic'.[229]

There have been exhaustive studies on the behaviors, and resultant stresses, of animals exposed to overcrowding. For instance, the population of Minnesota jackrabbits has been found to rise then crash at regular intervals. The common belief is that the deaths must be due to starvation. However, this is not the case. Food has been relatively abundant.

When autopsies were done on these rabbits, scientists found abnormalities in the liver and a state of *hypoglycemia* (low blood sugar) before the onset of death. They also found hemorrhages in the adrenals, thyroid and kidneys. These symptoms are typical of the chronic stress response affecting the hypothalamus-pituitary gland-adrenals axis (HPA Axis) mentioned in Chapter Four (page 71).[230]

On a small, 150-acre (0.6 km²) island off Chesapeake Bay, two deer were placed, and well fed and well taken care of. Yet when the population reached more than one deer every acre, a mysterious die-off began. Again, the adrenal stress response was found to be the primary cause.[231]

Before dying off from overpopulation, animals have been seen to display deviant behavior out of all proportion to what they would usually display if given adequate living space. The males displayed more aggressive behavior or went into an extreme reclusive mode, while females underwent spontaneous abortions and miscarriages, and infant mortality was much higher than normal.[232]

The conclusion from these studies is that somehow, when a population exceeds a level sustainable for the living space available, a process begins where the stress response is activated and death results for a significant portion of the population.

If human beings are essentially another link in the ecosystem, just like animals, can we conclude that the epidemic of disease currently afflicting us is a sign that we as a species have grown too populous for our own (and Earth's) good?

Here's my best guess. I mentioned before (Chapter Three, page 62) that consciousness is present in every living thing. It would then be fair to say that our planet is part of a higher-order system with a consciousness that encompasses all beings and things within Earth, just like our individual consciousness encompasses the germs living within our body.

Humanity may just be killing our host, planet Earth, with overpopulation. As I'm writing this (August 2016), the population of the world stands at 7.4 billion. An additional 78 million people are added to this population every year.[233]

We are decimating our rainforests, metaphorically the lungs of Gaia, to provide resources for humanity. As a result, animals and plants on Earth are going extinct at an unprecedented rate. Our soil is no longer being allowed to rest; a greater and greater strain is being placed every year to produce more and more food to feed all the hungry mouths.

Energy is critical to sustaining our living standards so oil and gas (metaphorically the blood of Earth) are being extracted for this purpose. As natural resources dwindle, we can expect that competition to gain access to these resources will be the basis for many wars and conflicts in the future.

No one probably said it better than Agent Smith in the movie Matrix (bolded text is mine):

*"I'd like to share a revelation that I've had during my time here. It came to me when I tried to classify your species and I realized that you aren't actually mammals. Every mammal on this planet instinctively develops a natural equilibrium with its surrounding environment, but you humans do not. You move to an area and you multiply and multiply until every natural resource is consumed, and the only way you can survive is to spread to another area. There is another organism on this planet that follows the same pattern. Do you know what it is? A virus. **Human beings are a disease, a cancer of this planet. You are a plague.** And we are the cure."*[234]

An analogy is probably fitting here. We often obsess over our weight; we just love losing those extra pounds. From our perspective, losing weight is a good thing. But those additional pounds have to be eliminated ('die') in order for us to have that slender figure. Similarly, if Earth is to detoxify, those cells (humans) that no longer serve the overall balance of the Earth's body have to be removed.

Overpopulation — and the response by Earth to bring the human population back to equilibrium — is then probably the underlying factor unconsciously pushing us as a species towards war and all kinds of depravities. This cascades, down the line, into traumas on the group and individual level, stress on the emotional and physical levels in the individual, and finally disease as we know it.

The problem of overpopulation of humanity is quoted as *The Last Taboo* by Mother Jones columnist Julia Whitty. She mentions that although scientists and politicians understand that this is the biggest problem on Earth today they keep silent because of the potential backlash from the public.[235]

Yet hiding from the problem does nothing to resolve it. My guess is that until we address the problem of overpopulation we'll not be able to resolve permanently the disease problems of humanity.

However, although we are all subjected to the Earth Soul's reaction to overpopulation, our individual soul consciousness determines how this reaction affects us personally.

Recall the Law of Attraction (Chapter Seven, page 122): the environment we attract is aligned with our consciousness. Since the traumas faced by each individual affect the Earth Soul, it is my hope that raising our individual consciousness, sometimes one individual at a time, through healing of these traumas will allow our species to grow in consciousness to solve the overpopulation issue collectively.

Ironically, it is the 'primitive' people of our ages that have been highlighting issues of ecology and sustainability since their exposure to 'civilized' people. For example, as early as 1854, Chief Seattle, a Native American leader from the US, says this:

"Humankind has not woven the web of life. We are but one thread within it. Whatever we do to the web, we do to ourselves. All things are bound together. All things are interconnected."[236]

Truly, we are interconnected and everything is just a reflection of the One Source. To be in balance with this One Source promises health; to be in conflict with it dooms us to disease.

Summary

The nature of our holographic universe means that there are self-similar systems at different levels of magnitude. Higher order systems tend to organize and control lower order systems. For example, living beings on Earth appear to have evolved based on cyclical galactic events.

Similarly, overpopulation of Earth by the human species has set off a compensatory mechanism by Gaia, the Earth Soul. The way humans have learnt to resolve the dilemma of more and more people competing for less and less resources is to engage in conflicts and war. The people involved in these conflicts, and their families, are then subjected to traumas and the resulting stress response in the body. This stress is then epigenetically transferred to descendants, ensuring that the population of humanity is brought back to balance with Earth through the mechanism of disease and premature death.

CONCLUSION — TMSD: How All Our Diseases are caused by Traumatic Memories

(TMSD, recall, is Traumatic Memories as Source of Disease.)

If you have ploughed your way through the book to this point, the conclusion, I congratulate you!

The concepts introduced in *Cracking The Disease Code* (CTDC) may well have been abstract or unfamiliar to readers brought up on a steady diet of mainstream medicine dogma. But I hope you will take the time to do further research on the studies and ideas brought up here (resources are provided after this Chapter). This will help you flesh out and answer questions on the true causes of disease, whether yours or those of people you care about.

Here's a summary of the vast ground we have covered in CTDC, and my answer to cracking the disease code:

There is a Source, and this is the highest-order system in our universe. The Source organizes and is responsible for all lower-order systems: the galaxy, our solar system, our Sun and Earth, and all living things within the Earth system.

A higher-order system organizes lower-order systems via morphogenetic fields. An individual morphogenetic field, or the individual soul, is part of the morphogenetic field of the family it belongs to, or the family soul, and so on and so forth to higher and higher orders of organization.

All events experienced by a lower-order system, say a human being, are stored as information we term 'memory' in the morphogenetic field of this individual; together, the memories of all the human beings in a family unit make up the morphogenetic field of the next higher-order system (the family soul).

The memories of all the families in a community make up the morphogenetic field of the community; the memories of all the communities in a region make up the morphogenetic field of the state; and so on. The morphogenetic field relating to The Source holds all the memories of every living thing, from every land and era, which has ever existed.

The Source is responsible for organizing all the physical and metabolic processes that take place in every one of us. If a person is able to perfectly access the information from the morphogenetic system of The Source then disease is not possible. In fact, not only disease but also misery, poverty, relationship problems — everything we do not want in our life — would all disappear if we are a complete vibrational match to The Source, because The Source is also the source of all joy, love and happiness.

Unfortunately, for almost all of us, we are not a complete vibrational match to The Source.

When we experience events, we also interpret and give meaning to these events. There are two basic ways we can interpret them — through the lens of Love or through the lens of Fear. Love and Fear are our two primary emotions, and all other emotions — courage, anger, sadness, frustration, etc — are merely different facets of these two emotions.

When our interpretation is based on Love, we make a Decision of Grace, and activate our parasympathetic system or the 'relaxation response'. When our interpretation is based on Fear, we make a Decision of Defeat, and activate our sympathetic system, or the

Conclusion

'stress response'. Therefore, the state of our health and life is actually dependent on the total amount of Love and Fear we have created in our life.

When we interpret an event with Fear or through a Decision of Defeat, trauma results, and the trauma memory is then stored in our morphogenetic field. Trauma memories act as blockages that prevent the information from a higher-order system from flowing into us.

Furthermore, these trauma memories, through resonance, attract similar events, creating a pattern in which we keep experiencing incidents that activate our usual pattern of feelings: abandonment, anger, betrayal, bitterness, envy, greed, hate, hopelessness, pride, resentment, sadness, etc.

The purpose of these events repeating in our life is to allow us to come to a new realization and decision about ourselves — that ultimately we are The Source and therefore that all our decisions should come from Love.

Traumatic memories are linked by association or resonance (depending on your perspective) in a COEX (Systems of Condensed Experiences) chain with the earliest memories being the most pivotal.

A trauma to an individual may have occurred in a past life. The Law of Attraction states that we will then be attracted to a family group with a similar pattern of emotions, and be reborn into this family to repeat this pattern of emotions. In Eastern traditions, this is known as *karma* (the Law of Cause and Effect: we reap what we sow).

Whilst in the womb and during birth, the traumas from our past lives and ancestral line get imprinted *physically* on us. For example (see Norbert's story, Chapter Ten, page 173), we experience birth traumas that are linked to earlier memories from our past life

Conclusion

so that by the time we are born we already have a certain personality. The idea that we are a clean slate at birth is not true.

These physical imprints (which are wired into our nervous system as well) make us more vulnerable than other people to experiencing certain emotions. You can experience the same event as someone else but feel different emotions, in different degrees, based on different imprints.

As we continue to experience childhood incidents of the same nature (drawn to us by the Law of Attraction), our vulnerabilities because of these imprints lead us to develop certain beliefs and make Decisions of Defeat that further ingrain these characteristics in us.

In addition, these vulnerabilities open us up to attachment by entities that are resonating with the same energies. These entities are hoping to complete their own 'unfinished business' through us.

By six years of age our personality has been essentially formed; it is the one we carry into adulthood. Changes to this personality structure are likely to be superficial rather than deep, no matter how much conscious effort we put into the effort, because the pillars of our personality reside mostly in our unconscious mind.

The traumatic memories we hold continuously trigger a stress response in us, resulting in the following typical sequence of events:

- The hypothalamus sends a signal to the pituitary gland that then signals the adrenals to pump out stress hormones like cortisol into our blood.
- Cortisol affects almost all the functions in our body. Our digestive system gets sluggish. Our adrenals become exhausted. The thyroid has to work harder because the thyroid hormone is now unable to get into the cells.

Conclusion

- We see first symptoms of hyperthyroidism, and then, when our thyroid becomes exhausted, a state of hypothyroidism.
- Without the thyroid hormone, cellular energy (known as ATP) is insufficient.
- Yeast is allowed to grow by the body as they help to produce energy through a secondary fermentation process.
- The body loses the ability to use energy for detoxification purposes.
- Toxins that we absorb from the environment cannot be eliminated from the system and have to be stored away safely.
- Inflammation is needed to kick-start elimination but over time, when the body becomes overwhelmed and inflammation fails, the toxins get deposited into the organs or in growths that may eventually turn cancerous.
- Inflammation gets ramped up even more (especially when cells become resistant to the influence of cortisol), leading to more pain and fatigue and deterioration of the organs.
- In this toxic environment, germs thrive. They are allowed by the body as clean-up crews to try to get the body functioning again, but at a cost: the germs also produce their own bio-toxins that the body has to deal with.
- At the DNA level, more biophotons are released to try to restore organization to our cells because we have 'tuned' ourselves out of the health template provided by The Source.

- Epigenetic changes also ensue, causing our genes to be switched on or off inappropriately, initiating the disease process.

Seen this way, disease is actually a process by which The Source can come to perfection through each of us. Since consciousness and the environment are really one and the same, we are both The Source out there in the universe as well as The Source in our body, via our cells ("As within, so without").

Our Higher Consciousness creates events to help us make either a decision of Love or a decision of Fear. If we choose to make a decision of Fear, The Source then sends us our next experience, asking us to choose again, in a continuing cycle until all of us come to a decision of Love at every moment.

When that happens, we would finally experience the truth — that we are The Source and Love — and fulfil the purpose of our human existence.

The logical question to ask is "Does all this mean that we should just accept our condition as it is?"

The answer is an emphatic 'No!' Since, as I've explained in CTDC, traumatic memories are the source of all disease, the logical thing to do is to deal with these traumatic memories to reverse our diseases. By doing this we are also helping higher-order systems like the Earth Soul since our individual traumas are stored as information there.

How we deal with these traumatic memories will be discussed in my next book, *Reversing the Disease Code*.

ABOUT THE AUTHOR

Darius Soon is Chief Practitioner of Radiant Wellness Centre, a wellness center he founded in 2011 in Singapore. He uses the energetic system he created, known as Medical Intuition System (MIS), to check the energy fields of his clients and do energy corrections for them. He also teaches his system to other healers so that they can become better healers. You can reach him at: www.RadiantWellnessCentre.com

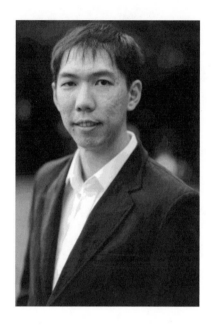

End Notes

Introduction

[1] Clarke, Roger (2012), A Natural History of Ghosts: 500 Years of Hunting for Proof, London: Particular Books, pp. 147 – 148

Chapter One

[2] Retrieved from scienceworld.wolfram.com/biography/Kelvin.html

[3] Powell, Diane Hennacy, M.D. (2009), The ESP Enigma, New York: Walker and Company, pp. 198.

[4] Tucker, Dr. Jim B. (2005), Life Before Life, A Scientific Investigation of Children's Memories of Previous Lives, New York: St. Martin's Press, Pp. 196.

[5] Greer, John Michael (2011), Monsters: An Investigator's Guide to Magical Beings, Woodbury, Minnesota: Llewellyn Publications, pp. 1.

[6] Radin, Dean, Ph.D (2013), Supernormal: Science, Yoga, and the Evidence for Extraordinary Psychic Abilities, New York: Random House/Deepak Chopra, pp. 58 – 59.

[7] Ibid, pp. 60.

[8] Rosenthal, R. (1976), Experimental Effects in Behavioural Research, John Wiley, New York.

[9] Church, Dawson, Ph.D. (2009), The Genie in your Genes, Nashville, Tennessee: Cumberland House Publishing, pp. 177.

[10] Evans, Dylan (2014), Placebo: Mind over Matter in Modern Medicine, New York: HarperCollins, pp. 35.

[11] Ibid, pp. 56.

[12] Ibid, pp. 270.

[13] Schlitz, Marilyn, PhD, and William Braud, PhD, Distant Intentionality and Healing: Assessing the Evidence (PDF), Retrieved from:
www.noetic.org/sites/default/files/uploads/files/DistantIntentionali ty.pdf

[14] For example, Bill Bengston has been conducting hands-on healing on rats in 14 controlled animal experiments over 6 different university laboratories. Retrieved from: bengstonresearch.com/research/scientific-articles. Of course, one can argue that animals, being sentient, can also be influenced by the placebo effect, and I would agree with that, because placebo effect is ultimately a phenomenon of the Mind, which is present in humans as well as animals.

Chapter Two

[15] Story of Royal Rife is retrieved from:
www.naturalnews.com/027104_cancer_WHO_Chi.html and educate-yourself.org/cn/rifetimelinemay1998.shtml

[16] The history of medicine is documented in Walker, Thomas (2004), The Force is with us: The Conspiracy against the Supernatural, Spiritual and Paranormal, Austin, Texas: Roaring Fork Limited, pp. 293-295.

[17] The story of AMA is documented in Bigelsen, Harvey MD with Lisa Haller (2011), Doctors are more harmful than germs – how surgery can be hazardous to your health – and what to do about it, Berkeley, California: North Atlantic Books, pp. 90.

[18] P.C. Gotzsche et al. (2007), Ghost authorship in Industry-initiated Randomised Trials, PloS Med, 2007; 4 (1): e19.

[19] Retrieved from: 247wallst.com/investing/2010/12/10/the-ten-worst-drug-recalls-in-the-history-of-the-fda/

[20] Gary Null et al., Death by Medicine, Life Extension Magazine (March 2004). Retrieved from: www.lifeextension.com/magazine/2004/3/awsi_death/Page-02

[21] Bland, Dr. Jeffrey S. (2015), The Disease Delusion: Conquering the Causes of Chronic Illness for a Healthier, Longer, and Happier Life, New York: Harper Wave, pp. 39.

[22] The concept of homotoxicology is covered in depth in Williams, Louisa L., M.S., D.C., N.D., (2011), Radical Medicine: Cutting-Edge Natural Therapies that Treats the Root Causes of Disease, Rochester, Vermont: Healing Arts Press, pg 18-21.

[23] Evans, Dylan (2014), Placebo: Mind over Matter in Modern Medicine, New York: HarperCollins, pp. 49.

[24] Ibid, pp. 49.

[25] Reardon, Sara (2014), "Gut-brain link grabs neuroscientists", Nature, 515, pg 175-177 (13 November 2014), Retrieved from www.nature.com/news/gut-brain-link-grabs-neuroscientists-1.16316

Chapter Three

[26] Tucker, Dr. Jim B. (2005), Life Before Life, A Scientific Investigation of Children's Memories of Previous Lives, New York: St. Martin's Press, Pp. 191 – 196.

[27] Wilcock, David (2012), Source Field Investigations: The Hidden Science and Lost Civilizations Behind the 2012 Prophecies, New York: Dutton, pp. 78.

[28] Powell, Diane Hennacy, M.D. (2009), The ESP Enigma, New York: Walker and Company, pp. 204 – 206.

[29] Ibid, pp. 204 – 206.

[30] Radin, Dean, Ph.D (2013), Supernormal: Science, Yoga, and the Evidence for Extraordinary Psychic Abilities, New York: Random House/Deepak Chopra, pp. 88 – 89.

[31] Refer to the Global Consciousness Project at global-mind.org/

[32] Radin, Dean, Ph.D (2013), Supernormal: Science, Yoga, and the Evidence for Extraordinary Psychic Abilities, New York: Random House/Deepak Chopra, pp. 91.

[33] Wilcock, David (2012), Source Field Investigations: The Hidden Science and Lost Civilizations Behind the 2012 Prophecies, New York: Dutton, pp. 36.

[34] The story of Nasruddin is retrieved from www.spiritual-minds.com/stories/mullah.htm

Chapter Four

[35] Leaky gut syndrome and associated symptoms are covered in Williams, Louisa L., M.S., D.C., N.D., (2011), Radical Medicine: Cutting-Edge Natural Therapies that Treats the Root Causes of Disease, Rochester, Vermont: Healing Arts Press, pg 232 - 243.

[36] Retrieved from adrenalfatigue.org/alcoholism-and-addiction/

[37] Langer, Stephen E., M.D., and James F. Scheer (2006), Solved: The Riddle of Illness, New York: McGraw-Hill Education, pp. 26.

[38] Ibid, pp. 50.

[39] Ibid, pp. 10.

[40] Ibid.

End Notes

[41] Horowitz, Richard I. (2013), Why Can't I Get Better? Solving the Mystery of Lyme and Chronic Disease, New York: St. Martin's Press, Pp. 279 - 280.

[42] Loyd, Alexander (2011), Healing Code: 6 Minutes to Heal the Source of your Health, Success or Relationship Issue, New York: Grand Central Life & Style, pp. 57.

[43] Mate, Gabor (2011), When the Body Says No: Exploring the Stress-Disease Connection, New Jersey: Wiley, pp. 32 - 34

[44] Horowitz, Richard I. (2013), Why Can't I Get Better? Solving the Mystery of Lyme and Chronic Disease, New York: St. Martin's Press, Pp. 387.

[45] Williams, Louisa L., M.S., D.C., N.D., (2011), Radical Medicine: Cutting-Edge Natural Therapies that Treats the Root Causes of Disease, Rochester, Vermont: Healing Arts Press, pg 240 - 241.

[46] Horowitz, Richard I. (2013), Why Can't I Get Better? Solving the Mystery of Lyme and Chronic Disease, New York: St. Martin's Press, Pp. 284 - 285.

[47] Langer, Stephen E., M.D., and James F. Scheer (2006), Solved: The Riddle of Illness, New York: McGraw-Hill Education, pp. 30.

[48] Horowitz, Richard I. (2013), Why Can't I Get Better? Solving the Mystery of Lyme and Chronic Disease, New York: St. Martin's Press, Pp. 279 - 280.

[49] Keown, Dr. Daniel, M.B. Ch.B, Lic. Ac (2014), The Spark in the Machine: How the Science of Acupuncture Explains the Mysteries of Western Medicine, London: Singing Dragon, pp. 144 – 148.

[50] Langer, Stephen E., M.D., and James F. Scheer (2006), Solved: The Riddle of Illness, New York: McGraw-Hill Education, pp. 134.

[51] Ibid, pp. 129.

[52] Mate, Gabor (2011), When the Body Says No: Exploring the Stress-Disease Connection, New Jersey: Wiley, pp. 35 – 36.

[53] Rankin, Dr. Lissa M.D. (2014), Mind Over Medicine: Scientific Proof That You Can Heal Yourself, Carksbad, California: Hay House, pp. 78.

[54] Horowitz, Richard I. (2013), Why Can't I Get Better? Solving the Mystery of Lyme and Chronic Disease, New York: St. Martin's Press, Pp. 284 - 285.

[55] Rankin, Dr. Lissa M.D. (2014), Mind Over Medicine: Scientific Proof That You Can Heal Yourself, Carksbad, California: Hay House, pp. 133 – 135.

[56] Horowitz, Richard I. (2013), Why Can't I Get Better? Solving the Mystery of Lyme and Chronic Disease, New York: St. Martin's Press, Pp. 284 - 285.

[57] Ibid.

[58] Mate, Gabor (2011), When the Body Says No: Exploring the Stress-Disease Connection, New Jersey: Wiley, pp. 32 – 34.

[59] Loyd, Alexander (2011), Healing Code: 6 Minutes to Heal the Source of your Health, Success or Relationship Issue, New York: Grand Central Life & Style, pp. 23.

Chapter Five

[60] Mate, Gabor (2011), When the Body Says No: Exploring the Stress-Disease Connection, New Jersey: Wiley, pp. 31.

[61] McLean, Paul (1990), The Triune Brain in Evolution: Role in Paleocelebral Functions, New York: Springer.

[62] Mate, Gabor (2011), When the Body Says No: Exploring the Stress-Disease Connection, New Jersey: Wiley, pp. 35 – 36.

[63] Ibid, pp. 32 – 34

[64] Levine, Peter A. (1997), Waking the Tiger: Healing Trauma, Berkeley, California: North Atlantic Books, pp. 15 - 21

[65] Mate, Gabor (2011), When the Body Says No: Exploring the Stress-Disease Connection, New Jersey: Wiley, pp. 32 - 34.

[66] Ibid, pp. 31

---

[67] Discussion of the Decision of Defeat can be found in Slavinski, Zivorad Mihajlovic (2005), Return to Oneness: Principles & Practice of Spiritual Technology, pp. 73 – 79.

[68] Mate, Gabor (2011), When the Body Says No: Exploring the Stress-Disease Connection, New Jersey: Wiley, pp. 86 - 87.

Chapter Six

[69] Bigelsen, Harvey MD with Lisa Haller (2011), Doctors are more harmful than germs – how surgery can be hazardous to your health – and what to do about it, Berkeley, California: North Atlantic Books, pp. 149 – 153.

[70] Church, Dawson, Ph.D. (2009), The Genie in your Genes, Nashville, Tennessee: Cumberland House Publishing, pp. 211.

[71] Loyd, Alexander (2011), Healing Code: 6 Minutes to Heal the Source of your Health, Success or Relationship Issue, New York: Grand Central Life & Style, pp. 24.

[72] Grof, Dr. Stanislav (1996), Realms of the Human Unconscious: Observations from LSD Research, London: Souvenir Press.

[73] Grof, Dr. Stanislav (2006), When the Impossible Happens: Adventures in Non-Ordinary Reality, Louisville, Colorado: Sounds True, pp. 280 – 282.

[74] Chamberlain, David (2013), Windows to the Womb: Revealing the Conscious Baby from Conception to Birth, Berkeley, California: North Atlantic Books, pp. 107 – 111.

[75] Grof, Dr. Stanislav (2006), When the Impossible Happens: Adventures in Non-Ordinary Reality, Louisville, Colorado: Sounds True, pp. 97.

[76] Verdult, Rien (2009), Caesarian Birth: Psychological Aspects in Babies, Journal of Prenatal and Perinatal Psychology and Medicine, 2009, 21,1/2, pg 29-41.

[77] Grof, Dr. Stanislav (2006), When the Impossible Happens: Adventures in Non-Ordinary Reality, Louisville, Colorado: Sounds True, pp. 97.

[78] Starecheski, Laura (2015), Can Family Secrets Make You Sick?, Retrieved from: www.npr.org/sections/health-shots/2015/03/02/377569413/can-family-secrets-make-you-sick

[79] Retrieved from: www.cdc.gov/violenceprevention/acestudy/findings.html

[80] Mate, Gabor (2011), When the Body Says No: Exploring the Stress-Disease Connection, New Jersey: Wiley, pp. 16.

[81] Slavinski, Zivorad (2007), PEAT: Primordial Energy Activation and Transcendence and the Neutralization of Polarities, Arelena Publishing, pp. 33.

[82] Church, Dawson, Ph.D. (2009), The Genie in your Genes, Nashville, Tennessee: Cumberland House Publishing, pp. 74.

Chapter Seven

[83] Sylvia, Claire (2008), I was given a young man's heart - and started craving beer and Kentucky Fried Chicken. My daughter said I even walked like a man, Daily Mail, 9 April 2008, retrieved from: www.dailymail.co.uk/health/article-558256/I-given-young-mans-heart---started-craving-beer-Kentucky-Fried-Chicken-My-daughter-said-I-walked-like-man.html

[84] Sheldrake, Rupert (2012), The Science Delusion: Freeing the Spirit of Enquiry, Philadelphia, Pennsylvania: Coronet, pp. 190.

[85] Ibid, pp. 193.

[86] Walker, Thomas (2004), The Force is with us: The Conspiracy against the Supernatural, Spiritual and Paranormal, Austin, Texas: Roaring Fork Limited, pp. 92 – 93.

[87] Zolfagharifard, Ellie (2015), Are we living in a hologram? For the first time, scientists prove strange theory could be true in 'realistic models' of our universe, Daily Mail, 27 April 2015, Retrieved from: www.dailymail.co.uk/sciencetech/article-3057957/Are-living-HOLOGRAM-time-scientists-prove-strange-theory-true-realistic-models-universe.html

End Notes

[88] Lockhart, Maureen Ph.D. (2010), The Subtle Energy Body: The Complete Guide, Vermont: Inner Traditions, pp. 57 - 59.

[89] Conner, Steve (2015), Single DNA Molecule Could Store Information for a Million Years Following Scientific Breakthrough, Independent, 18 April 2015, retrieved from: www.independent.co.uk/news/science/single-dna-molecule-could-store-information-for-a-million-years-following-scientific-breakthrough-10459560.html

[90] Powell, Diane Hennacy, M.D. (2009), The ESP Enigma, New York: Walker and Company, pp. 212 - 213.

[91] Sheldrake, Rupert (2012), The Science Delusion: Freeing the Spirit of Enquiry, Philadelphia, Pennsylvania: Coronet, pp. 207.

[92] Ibid, pp. 208.

[93] Powell, Diane Hennacy, M.D. (2009), The ESP Enigma, New York: Walker and Company, pp. 177 - 178.

[94] Ibid.

[95] Sheldrake, Rupert (2012), The Science Delusion: Freeing the Spirit of Enquiry, Philadelphia, Pennsylvania: Coronet, pp. 99.

[96] Wilcock, David (2012), Source Field Investigations: The Hidden Science and Lost Civilizations Behind the 2012 Prophecies, New York: Dutton, pp. 167 - 171.

[97] Klinghardt, Dietrich, M.D., Ph.D, Autonomic Response Testing I, Seattle: Klinghardt Academy, pp. 21.

[98] Ibid.

[99] Ibid, pp. 75 – 78.

[100] Sheldrake, Rupert (2012), The Science Delusion: Freeing the Spirit of Enquiry, Philadelphia, Pennsylvania: Coronet, pp. 179.

Chapter Eight

[101] Retrieved from: www.genome.gov/10001356

[102] Wilcock, David (2012), Source Field Investigations: The Hidden Science and Lost Civilizations Behind the 2012 Prophecies, New York: Dutton, pp. 198.

[103] Sheldrake, Rupert (2012), The Science Delusion: Freeing the Spirit of Enquiry, Philadelphia, Pennsylvania: Coronet, pp. 168.

[104] Ibid.

[105] Ibid.

[106] Church, Dawson, Ph.D. (2009), The Genie in your Genes, Nashville, Tennessee: Cumberland House Publishing, pp. 35.

[107] Horowitz, Richard I. (2013), Why Can't I Get Better? Solving the Mystery of Lyme and Chronic Disease, New York: St. Martin's Press, Pp. 249 – 250.

[108] Free, Wynn (2004), The Reincarnation of Edgar Cayce: Interdimensional Communication and Global Transformation, Mumbai: Frog Books, pp. 344 – 346.

[109] Church, Dawson, Ph.D. (2009), The Genie in your Genes, Nashville, Tennessee: Cumberland House Publishing, pp. 44 - 47.

[110] Free, Wynn (2004), The Reincarnation of Edgar Cayce: Interdimensional Communication and Global Transformation, Mumbai: Frog Books, pp. 344 – 346.

[111] The usefulness of junk DNA are detailed in Park, Alice (2012), Junk DNA Not So Useless After All, Time Magazine, 6 Sep 2012, retrieved from: healthland.time.com/2012/09/06/junk-dna-not-so-useless-after-all/

[112] Ibid.

[113] Church, Dawson, Ph.D. (2009), The Genie in your Genes, Nashville, Tennessee: Cumberland House Publishing, pp. 44 - 47.

[114] Ibid.

[115] Petronis, A. (2010), 'Epigenetics as a unifying principle in the aetiology of complex traits and diseases', Nature, 465, 721 - 7 and Harmon, Katherine (2012), Junk DNA Holds Clues to Common Diseases, Scientific American, 5 Sep 2012, retrieved from: www.scientificamerican.com/article/junk-dna-encode/

[116] Wilcock, David (2012), Source Field Investigations: The Hidden Science and Lost Civilizations Behind the 2012 Prophecies, New York: Dutton, pp. 160 - 164.

[117] Ibid, pp. 176.

[118] Ibid, pp. 176 - 177.

[119] Ibid, pp. 177 - 178.

[120] Ibid, pp. 209.

[121] Ibid, pp. 206 - 207.

[122] Ibid, pp. 198 - 199.

Chapter Nine

[123] Carey, Nessey (2013), The Epigenetics Revolution: How Modern Biology is Rewriting our Understanding of Genetics, Disease and Inheritance, New York: Columbia University Press, pp. 2 - 4.

[124] Francis, Richard C. (2012), Epigenetics: How Environment Shapes Our Genes, New York: W. W. Norton & Company, pp. 86

[125] McTaggart, Lynn (2011), The Bond: Connecting through the Space between Us, New York: Simon & Schuster, pp. 21 - 22

[126] Ibid.

[127] Carey, Nessey (2013), The Epigenetics Revolution: How Modern Biology is Rewriting our Understanding of Genetics, Disease and Inheritance, New York: Columbia University Press, pp. 5.

[128] Ibid, pp. 242 - 243.

[129] Carey, Nessey (2013), The Epigenetics Revolution: How Modern Biology is Rewriting our Understanding of Genetics, Disease and Inheritance, New York: Columbia University Press, pp. 63.

[130] Schutzenbenger, Anne Ancelin (1998), The Ancestor Syndrome: Transgenerational Psychotherapy and the Hidden Links in the Family Tree, Abingdon-and-Thames: Routledge, pp. 58.

[131] Ibid, pp. 17 - 25.

[132] Hellinger, Bert (1998), Love's Hidden Symmetry: What Makes Love Work in Relationships, Phoenix, Arizona: Zeig, Tucker & Theisen, pp. 111 - 112.

[133] Ibid, pp. 153.

[134] Ibid, pp. 115 - 116.

[135] Sullivan, Natalia O' and Nicola Grayden (2013), The Ancestral Continuum: Unlock the Secrets of Who You Really Are, New York: Simon & Schuster, pp. 115.

[136] Boklage, C.E. (1995). "Chapter 4:The frequency and survivability of natural twin conceptions". In Keith, Louis G.; Papiernik, Emile; et al. Multiple Pregnancy: Epidemiology, Gestation and Perinatal Outcome (1st ed.), New York: Taylor & Francis Group. pp. 41-2, 49.

[137] Sullivan, Natalia O' and Nicola Grayden (2013), The Ancestral Continuum: Unlock the Secrets of Who You Really Are, New York: Simon & Schuster, pp. 115 - 120.

[138] Ibid, pp. 119.

[139] Sullivan, Natalia O' and Nicola Grayden (2013), The Ancestral Continuum: Unlock the Secrets of Who You Really Are, New York: Simon & Schuster, pp. 135.

[140] Hellinger, Bert (1998), Love's Hidden Symmetry: What Makes Love Work in Relationships, Phoenix, Arizona: Zeig, Tucker & Theisen, pp. 153.

[141] Sullivan, Natalia O' and Nicola Grayden (2013), The Ancestral Continuum: Unlock the Secrets of Who You Really Are, New York: Simon & Schuster, pp. 152.

[142] Thomson, Helen (2015), Study of Holocaust Survivors finds Trauma passed on to Children's Genes, The Guardian, 21 Aug 2015, retrieved from: www.theguardian.com/science/2015/aug/21/study-of-holocaust-survivors-finds-trauma-passed-on-to-childrens-genes

[143] Free, Wynn (2004), The Reincarnation of Edgar Cayce: Interdimensional Communication and Global Transformation, Mumbai: Frog Books, pp. 344 – 346.

[144] Sullivan, Natalia O' and Nicola Grayden (2013), The Ancestral Continuum: Unlock the Secrets of Who You Really Are, New York: Simon & Schuster, pp. 267.

[145] Numbers 14:18

Chapter Ten

[146] Tucker, Dr. Jim B. (2005), Life Before Life, A Scientific Investigation of Children's Memories of Previous Lives, New York: St. Martin's Press, Pp. 114 – 116.

[147] Ibid, pp. 52.

---

[148] Walker, Thomas (2004), The Force is with us: The Conspiracy against the Supernatural, Spiritual and Paranormal, Austin, Texas: Roaring Fork Limited, pp. 172 - 175.

[149] Ibid.

[150] Flanagan, Bob (2015), Indian Researchers Prove Reality of Reincarnation, World News Daily Report, 16 Feb 2015, retrieved from: worldnewsdailyreport.com/indian-researchers-prove-reality-of-reincarnation/

[151] Grof, Dr. Stanislav (2006), When the Impossible Happens: Adventures in Non-Ordinary Reality, Louisville, Colorado: Sounds True, pp. 137.

[152] Walker, Thomas (2004), The Force is with us: The Conspiracy against the Supernatural, Spiritual and Paranormal, Austin, Texas: Roaring Fork Limited, pp. 175.

[153] Grof, Dr. Stanislav (2006), When the Impossible Happens: Adventures in Non-Ordinary Reality, Louisville, Colorado: Sounds True, pp. 280 - 282.

Chapter Eleven

[154] Marohn, Stephanie (2003), The Natural Medicine Guide to Schizophrenia, Newburyport, Massachusetts: Hampton Roads Publishing Company, pp. 178 - 189.

[155] Modi, Shakuntala (1998), Remarkable Healings: A Psychiatrist Discovers Unsuspected Roots of Mental and Physical Illnesses, Newburyport, Massachusetts: Hampton Roads Publishing Company, pp. 35 - 38.

[156] Wickland, Dr. Carl A. (2014), Thirty Years Among the Dead: Obsessions and "Curses" Removed through the Work of the Medium Mrs Wickland, New Brunswirk, New Jersey: Inner Light.

[157] Spiegel, Lee (2013), Spooky Number of Americans Believe in Ghosts, Huffington Post, 2 Feb 2013, retrieved from: www.huffingtonpost.com/2013/02/02/real-ghosts-americans-poll_n_2049485.html

[158] Retrieved from: www.pewresearch.org/fact-tank/2015/10/30/18-of-americans-say-theyve-seen-a-ghost/

[159] Roland, Paul (2012), Ghosts: An Exploration of the Spiritual World, from Apparitions to Haunted Places, London: Arcturus, pp. 15.

[160] Read the book by Schwartz, Gary E. (2003), The Afterlife Experiments: Breakthrough Scientific Evidence of Life After Death, New York: Atria Books.

[161] Spiegel, Lee (2013), Life After Death Project: Forrest J Ackerman's Friends Claim He's Speaking To Them From The Dead, Huffington Post, 17 May 2013, retrieved from: www.huffingtonpost.com/2013/05/17/life-after-death-project-forest-j-ackerman_n_3280368.html

[162] Roland, Paul (2012), Ghosts: An Exploration of the Spiritual World, from Apparitions to Haunted Places, London: Arcturus, pp. 15.

[163] Ibid, pp. 22 – 25.

[164] First and Second Deaths are discussed in Greer, John Michael (2011), Monsters: An Investigator's Guide to Magical Beings, Woodbury, Minnesota: Llewellyn Publications, pp. 21.

[165] Ibid.

[166] Retrieved from: www.soul-guidance.com/houseofthesun/spirits.htm

[167] Modi, Shakuntala (1998), Remarkable Healings: A Psychiatrist Discovers Unsuspected Roots of Mental and Physical Illnesses, Newburyport, Massachusetts: Hampton Roads Publishing Company, pp. 578.

[168] Retrieved from: www.soul-guidance.com/houseofthesun/spirits.htm

[169] Marohn, Stephanie (2003), The Natural Medicine Guide to Schizophrenia, Newburyport, Massachusetts: Hampton Roads Publishing Company, pp. 178 – 189.

---

[170] Nested entities are discussed in Baldwin, William J. (1995), Spirit Releasement Therapy: A Technique Manual, 2nd Edition, London: Headline Books, pp. 307 – 313.

[171] Retrieved from: www.soul-guidance.com/houseofthesun/spirits.htm

[172] Ibid.

[173] Wallace, Charles P. (1990), Mysterious Ailment Takes Heavy Toll Among Thais : Southeast Asia: The Sudden Unexplained Nocturnal Death Syndrome has killed hundreds of young men. Doctors remain baffled, Los Angeles Times, 23 Mar 1990, Retrieved from: articles.latimes.com/1990-03-23/news/mn-715_1_sudden-unexplained-nocturnal-death-syndrome

[174] The story of Hmong and SUNDS is found in Greer, John Michael (2011), Monsters: An Investigator's Guide to Magical Beings, Woodbury, Minnesota: Llewellyn Publications, pp. 15 – 19.

[175] Shamans believed in three causes of illness – power loss, soul loss and intrusion by spirits. These three are correlated: the presence of power loss and soul loss allows a void for the spirits to enter into the energy field of the person. Therefore the statement that 100 percent of illnesses are caused by spirits is a simplification of a more complicated process which would be elaborated further when we put all the ideas together in the conclusion. For a deeper discussion of this topic from the perspective of shamans, read

www.sandraingerman.com/sandrasarticles/abstractonshamanism.ht
ml

Chapter Twelve

[176] Retrieved from en.wikipedia.org/wiki/Alexander_Fleming

[177] Bigelsen, Harvey MD with Lisa Haller (2011), Doctors are more
harmful than germs – how surgery can be hazardous to your health –
and what to do about it, Berkeley, California: North Atlantic Books,
pp. 83.

[178] Ibid, pp. 83 – 87.

[179] Walker, Thomas (2004), The Force is with us: The Conspiracy
against the Supernatural, Spiritual and Paranormal, Austin, Texas:
Roaring Fork Limited, pp. 420 - 421.

[180] Ibid.

[181] Retrieved from www.whale.to/v/rife.html.

[182] Bigelsen, Harvey MD with Lisa Haller (2011), Doctors are more
harmful than germs – how surgery can be hazardous to your health –
and what to do about it, Berkeley, California: North Atlantic Books,
pp. 164.

[183] Evans, Dylan (2014), Placebo: Mind over Matter in Modern
Medicine, New York: HarperCollins, pp. 135.

[184] Bigelsen, Harvey MD with Lisa Haller (2011), Doctors are more harmful than germs – how surgery can be hazardous to your health – and what to do about it, Berkeley, California: North Atlantic Books, pp. 83 - 87.

[185] Retrieved from: lymediseaseresource.com/wordpress/chronic-lyme-disease-or-mercury-poisoning/

[186] Credit should be given to Dr. Dietrich Klinghardt, M.D. who talks about this link in the Autonomic Response Testing (ART) III class that I went to.

[187] Refer to books like: Yoseph, James and Hannah (2014), Proof for the Cancer-Fungus Connection: And What You Can Do to Prevent and Cure Cancer, Hannah Yoseph and Simoncini, Dr. T. (2007), Cancer is a Fungus: A Revolution in Tumour Therapy, Milan: Edizioni

[188] Williams, Louisa L., M.S., D.C., N.D., (2011), Radical Medicine: Cutting-Edge Natural Therapies that Treats the Root Causes of Disease, Rochester, Vermont: Healing Arts Press, pp. 71.

[189] Retrieved from: moldvictim.org/sick-building-syndrome/

[190] Williams, Louisa L., M.S., D.C., N.D., (2011), Radical Medicine: Cutting-Edge Natural Therapies that Treats the Root Causes of Disease, Rochester, Vermont: Healing Arts Press, pp. 57.

[191] Ibid, pp. 71.

[192] Ibid.

[193] Ibid, pp. 60 – 61.

[194] Mercury Policy Project (2011), WHO Report Suggests "Phase Down" of Dental Amalgam Globally; Breakthrough Will Lead to Phase Out of Dental Mercury, Say NGOs, retrieved from: www.prnewswire.com/news-releases/who-report-suggests-phase-down-of-dental-amalgam-globally-breakthrough-will-lead-to-phase-out-of-dental-mercury-say-ngos-131548538.html

[195] Williams, Louisa L., M.S., D.C., N.D., (2011), Radical Medicine: Cutting-Edge Natural Therapies that Treats the Root Causes of Disease, Rochester, Vermont: Healing Arts Press, pp. 450.

[196] Ibid, pp. 452.

[197] Klinghardt, Dietrich, M.D., Ph.D, Autonomic Response Testing I, Seattle: Klinghardt Academy, pp. 78.

[198] Horowitz, Richard I. (2013), Why Can't I Get Better? Solving the Mystery of Lyme and Chronic Disease, New York: St. Martin's Press, Pp. 222 - 223.

[199] Ibid, pp. 392.

[200] Sheldrake, Rupert (2012), The Science Delusion: Freeing the Spirit of Enquiry, Philadelphia, Pennsylvania: Coronet, pp. 175.

Chapter Thirteen

[201] Read Hartmann, Thom (2001), The Last Hours of Ancient Sunlight: Waking Up to Personal and Global Transformation, London: Hodder Paperback.

[202] Cousens, Gabriel (2000), Conscious Eating, Berkeley, California: North Atlantic Books, pp. 577

[203] Read Druker, Steven (2015), Altered Genes, Twisted Truth: How the Venture to Genetically Engineer Our Food Has Subverted Science, Corrupted Government, and Systematically Deceived the Public, Clear River Press.

[204] Cousens, Gabriel (2000), Conscious Eating, Berkeley, California: North Atlantic Books, pp. 577

[205] Retrieved from: articles.mercola.com/sites/articles/archive/2011/08/21/enzymes-special-report.aspx

[206] Santarelli, R. L., Pierre, F., & Corpet, D. E. (2008), Processed meat and colorectal cancer: a review of epidemiologic and experimental evidence, Nutrition and Cancer, 60(2), 131–144. doi.org/10.1080/01635580701684872

[207] Williams, Louisa L., M.S., D.C., N.D., (2011), Radical Medicine: Cutting-Edge Natural Therapies that Treats the Root Causes of Disease, Rochester, Vermont: Healing Arts Press, pp. 169.

[208] Read Wolcott, William L. and Trish Fahey (2002), The Metabolic Typing Diet: Customize Your Diet To: Free Yourself from Food Cravings: Achieve Your Ideal Weight; Enjoy High Energy and Robust Health; Prevent and Reverse Disease, New York: Harmony.

[209] Horowitz, Richard I. (2013), Why Can't I Get Better? Solving the Mystery of Lyme and Chronic Disease, New York: St. Martin's Press, Pp. 371 - 373.

[210] Williams, Louisa L., M.S., D.C., N.D., (2011), Radical Medicine: Cutting-Edge Natural Therapies that Treats the Root Causes of Disease, Rochester, Vermont: Healing Arts Press, pp. 233.

[211] Others have come to similar conclusions. See Ibid, pp. 202.

[212] Servick, Kelly (2013), How Exercise Beefs Up the Brain, Science, 10 Oct 2013, retrieved from: www.sciencemag.org/news/2013/10/how-exercise-beefs-brain

Chapter Fourteen

[213] McTaggart, Lynn (2011), The Bond: Connecting through the Space between Us, New York: Simon & Schuster, pp. 37.

[214] Ibid, pp. 46.

[215] Ibid, pp. 40.

[216] Ibid, pp. 39.

[217] Ibid, pp. 42 – 44.

[218] Retrieved from: blacktolife.com/biophotonics/

[219] Church, Dawson, Ph.D. (2009), The Genie in your Genes, Nashville, Tennessee: Cumberland House Publishing, pp. 124.

[220] Retrieved from: www.earthbreathing.co.uk/sr.htm

[221] Ulrike Banis, MD, author of Geopathic Stress - and What You Can Do About It reports, "my experience - being a medical professional myself - is that at least 30 percent of all chronic medical conditions are derived from this cause - or to put it differently, our patients would be, on average, 30 percent healthier if we manage to find good sleeping places for everyone." Retrieved from: www.geopathology.com/geopathology-articles/Ulrike-Banis.pdf

From 1953 to 1993, Dr. Ernst Hartmann, MD, found all cases of cancer being linked to geopathic stress. Austrian teacher and dowser Käthe Bachler dowsed 3000 sleeping locations over 14 countries and found geopathic stress to be responsible for all cases of cancer she saw. Retrieved from: www.healingcancernaturally.com/geopathic-stress-and-cancer.html

[222] Walker, Thomas (2004), The Force is with us: The Conspiracy against the Supernatural, Spiritual and Paranormal, Austin, Texas: Roaring Fork Limited, pp. 288 - 289.

Chapter Fifteen

[223] Raup, DM; Sepkoski Jr, JJ (1984). "Periodicity of Extinctions in the Geological Past". Proceedings of the National Academy of Sciences of the United States of America 81 (3): 801–5 and Rohde, R.; Muller, R. (2005). "Cycles in fossil diversity". Nature 434 (7030): 208–210.

[224] Free, Wynn (2004), The Reincarnation of Edgar Cayce: Interdimensional Communication and Global Transformation, Mumbai: Frog Books, pp. 398.

[225] Retrieved from en.wikipedia.org/wiki/Emerald_Tablet

[226] Koestler, Arthur (1982), The Ghost in the Machine, Last Century Media, pp. 48.

[227] See Baryshev, Yurij and Pekka Teerikorpi (2002), Discovery of Cosmic Fractals, World Scientific Pub Co Inc. On the other hand, there has also been some research that has shown that the universe is not a fractal, for example see: www.newscientist.com/article/dn22214-giant-fractals-are-out-the-universe-is-a-big-smoothie/. So it seems like there's still no definitive answer.

[228] Lovelock, James (2000), Gaia: A New Look at Life on Earth, Oxford: Oxford University Press.

[229] Hoagland, Hudson (1964), "Cybernetics of Population Control", Bulletin of the Atomic Scientists, Vol 2, Issue 2

[230] Ibid.

[231] Ibid.

[232] Ibid.

[233] Retrieved from: www.worldometers.info/world-population/

[234] Retrieved from: www.imdb.com/character/ch0000745/quotes

[235] Retrieved from: www.motherjones.com/environment/2010/05/population-growth-india-vatican?page=1

[236] O'Sullivan, Natalia and Nicola Grayden (2013), The Ancestral Continuum: Unlock the Secrets of Who You Really Are, New York: Simon & Schuster, pp. 265.